Advanced Resuscitation of the Newborn Infant

2nd Edition, May 2021

Reprinted June 2022

ARNI

Advanced Resuscitation of the Newborn Infant
2nd Edition, May 2021

Reprinted June 2022

ISBN 978-1-903812-40-2

Copyright © Resuscitation Council UK, 2021.

All rights reserved. No part of this publication may be reproduced or transmitted in any form or by any means, electronic, mechanical, photocopying, recording, or otherwise without the prior written permission of Resuscitation Council UK (RCUK). Permission must also be obtained before any part of this publication is stored in any information storage or retrieval system of any nature.

Published by © Resuscitation Council UK 2021
5th Floor, Tavistock House North, Tavistock Square, London WC1H 9HR
Tel: 020 7388 4678 email: enquiries@resus.org.uk www.resus.org.uk

Printed by All About Print.
Tel: 020 7205 4022 email: hello@allaboutprint.co.uk www.allaboutprint.co.uk
Printed on responsibly sourced environmentally friendly paper made with elemental chlorine free fibre from legal and sustainably managed forests.

Photographs © Resuscitation Council UK

Photography by Ed Tyler and Ashley Prytherch
Colour plates reproduced with permission of the Northern Neonatal Network who retain copyright.

Design and artwork by Fruition London
www.fruitionlondon.com

The Resuscitation Council UK guidelines are adapted from the European Resuscitation Council guidelines and have been developed using a process accredited by The National Institute for Health and Care Excellence. The UK guidelines are consistent with the European guidelines but include minor modifications to reflect the needs of the National Health Service.

This Advanced Resuscitation of the Newborn Infant (ARNI) manual is written by Resuscitation Council UK ARNI Subcommittee and forms part of the resources for Resuscitation Council UK ARNI course, which is delivered in accredited course centres throughout the UK.

Acknowledgements

We would like to acknowledge the ARNI Subcommittee who all contributed to the development of this manual and the ARNI course. In particular we would like to thank Professor Jonathan Wyllie who was the inaugural chair of the ARNI Subcommittee. Thank you to BLISS without whose support the development of the ARNI course and manual would not have been possible. We also acknowledge Dr. Sean Ainsworth for his substantial help with the manuscript and the contributions of Professor Dennis Azzopardi, Dr. Nick Archer and Dr. Jane Gill.

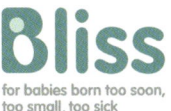

We would like to thank the parents who consented to pictures of their baby being used in ARNI materials, including Hazel Khodabocus for the drawing of her daughter.

We would like to acknowledge the work of colleagues in the global resuscitation community especially the work of the International Liaison Committee on Resuscitation and the European Resuscitation Council.

We would like to thank the British Association of Perinatal Medicine for permission to reproduce the Managing the Difficult Airway in the Neonate escalation policy and the Neonatal Early Warning Score (NEWS) Chart.

We thank the Nuffield Hospital, Guildford, for the use of their facilities, The Royal Surrey County Hospital NHS Foundation Trust, specifically the Resuscitation Department for their assistance with photography, Lifecast Body Simulation for the loan of manikins and all the Instructors who gave up their time to take part in the photography shoot.

We thank Ed Tyler and Ashley Prytherch for the photography taken and for being digitally prepared for the manual.

Editors

Joe Fawke
Jonathan Cusack

Core editorial group

Joe Fawke
Sean Ainsworth
Adam Benson Clarke
Jonathan Cusack
Isabelle Hamilton-Bower
Sue Hampshire
John Madar
Vix Monnelly
Jonathan Wyllie

Contributors

Louise Anthony
Charlotte Bennett
Adam Benson Clarke
Caroline Buckley
Clare Cane
Andrew Coleman
Jonathan Cusack
Bethan Dean
Joe Fawke
Ruth Gottstein
Isabelle Hamilton-Bower
Sue Hampshire
Ita Kelly
Tng Kwok
Cassie Lawn
Kevin Mackie
John Madar
Nicky McCarthy
Vix Monnelly
Clare Morfoot
Lidia Tyszczuk
Vivienne van Someren
Fiona Wood
Jonathan Wyllie
Jenny Ziprin

Contents

01 **Introduction to the course** ... 7
   Aims of ARNI ... 7
   Learning outcomes ... 7
   The ARNI approach ... 8
   Assessment on the ARNI Course ... 8
   Why is ARNI needed? ... 8
   Science and guidelines ... 10
   Further reading ... 10

02 **Resuscitation at birth** ... 11
   Introduction ... 11
   Preparation ... 12
   Umbilical cord management ... 12
   Delayed cord clamping ... 12
   After delivery ... 15
   Stimulation ... 15
   Pulse oximetry ... 15
   More complex resuscitation situations ... 18
   When to stop resuscitation ... 18
   Transferring to the neonatal unit ... 18
   Early postnatal management priorities ... 19
   Further reading ... 20

03 **Management of extreme prematurity** ... 21
   Introduction ... 21
   Antenatal care ... 21
   Antenatal counselling ... 22
   Preparation and planning ... 22
   Dealing with the extremely preterm baby at birth ... 22
   Surfactant ... 23
   Early care of the extremely preterm infant ... 24
   Progress and prognosis ... 25
   Further reading ... 27

04 **Recognition of the deteriorating infant** ... 29
   Introduction ... 29
   Situational awareness ... 30
   Neonatal early warning scores (NEWS) ... 30
   Interpretation ... 30
   Early effective intervention ... 32
   Initial rapid clinical assessment ... 32
   Interpreting observations and managing problems ... 33
   Putting it all together – interpretation with initial action ... 36
   Life-threatening features ... 36
   Further ABCDEF assessment ... 36
   Calling for help ... 36
   Further reading ... 38

05 **Communication, human factors and team working** ... 39
   Introduction ... 39
   SBAR – a structured communication tool ... 40
   Human factors ... 40
   Systems ... 40
   Processes ... 41
   Procedures ... 41
   Team working, human behaviours and abilities ... 41
   Errors and being wrong ... 44
   Rehearsal ... 44
   Further reading ... 46

06 **Communicating with families** ... 47
   Introduction ... 47
   Principles of effective communication with families ... 48
   Presence of parents during resuscitation ... 48
   When to stop resuscitation ... 48
   Antenatal counselling for extremely preterm birth ... 48
   Unsuccessful resuscitation ... 49
   Organ donation ... 50
   Further reading ... 52

07 **Advanced airway management** ... 53
   Introduction ... 53
   Airway opening manoeuvres ... 54
   Airway opening adjuncts ... 55
   Oxygen delivery systems ... 56
   ARNI course face mask ventilation station ... 58
   Methods of assisted ventilation ... 60
   Tracheal intubation ... 61
   Anatomical considerations ... 61
   Verification of tracheal tube placement ... 63
   End-tidal CO_2 detection ... 63
   Management of the difficult airway – maintaining a safe approach ... 63
   'Can't intubate, can't ventilate' ... 65
   Further reading ... 66

08 **Cardiovascular problems** ... 67
   Introduction ... 67
   The cyanotic baby ... 68
   The hyperoxia test ... 69
   Duct dependent congenital heart disease – physiology, recognition and management ... 69
   Persistent pulmonary hypertension of the newborn infant ... 71
   Heart failure in the newborn infant ... 71
   Neonatal arrhythmias ... 72
   Atrial flutter ... 73
   Complete heart block ... 73
   The hypotensive infant ... 74
   Inotropes ... 74
   Further reading ... 76

Contents

09 Neonatal surgical conditions **77**
    Introduction 77
    Tracheoesophageal fistula and oesophageal atresia 78
    Duodenal atresia 78
    Ischaemic bowel and volvulus 79
    Abdominal wall defects: Gastroschisis and Exomphalos 79
    Congenital diaphragmatic hernia (CDH) 80
    Spina bifida/myelomeningocoele 80
    Necrotising enterocolitis 81
    Further reading 84

10 Sepsis **85**
    Introduction 85
    Long term outcomes 85
    Pathogens 86
    Early onset neonatal infection 86
    Late onset neonatal infection 87
    Differential diagnosis 88
    Managing a baby with signs of neonatal sepsis 88
    Further investigations 89
    Treatment of infection 89
    Further reading 90

11 Neonatal encephalopathy **91**
    Introduction 91
    Hypoxic ischaemic encephalopathy (HIE) 92
    Clinical management on the neonatal unit 93
    Information gathering and documentation 93
    Neurological monitoring 93
    Cerebral function monitoring (CFM) 94
    Cranial ultrasound scanning 96
    Magnetic resonance imaging 96
    Therapeutic hypothermia 96
    Prognosis 98
    Focal cerebral infarction 99
    Subgaleal haemorrhage 99
    Infection and metabolic disturbances 99
    Further reading 100

12 Unexpected problems in the term infant **101**
    Introduction 101
    Sudden unexpected postnatal collapse (SUPC) 102
    Hypoglycaemia 104
    The blue or grey baby 105
    Sepsis 106
    Seizures 106
    Further reading 108

13 Practical procedures **109**
    Introduction 109
    Infection prevention 109
    Neonatal percutaneous central line insertion (long line) 110
    Insertion of an intraosseous line 110
    Umbilical line insertion 111
    Peripheral arterial line insertion 111
    Seldinger chest drain insertion 112
    Surgical chest drain insertion 114
    Emergency needle thoracocentesis 115
    Lumbar puncture (LP) 116
    Further reading 117

Appendices **118**
    A   Interpreting blood gases 119
    B   Three key ways to reduce mask leak 122
    C   Personal protective equipment (PPE) 123

Useful links 124

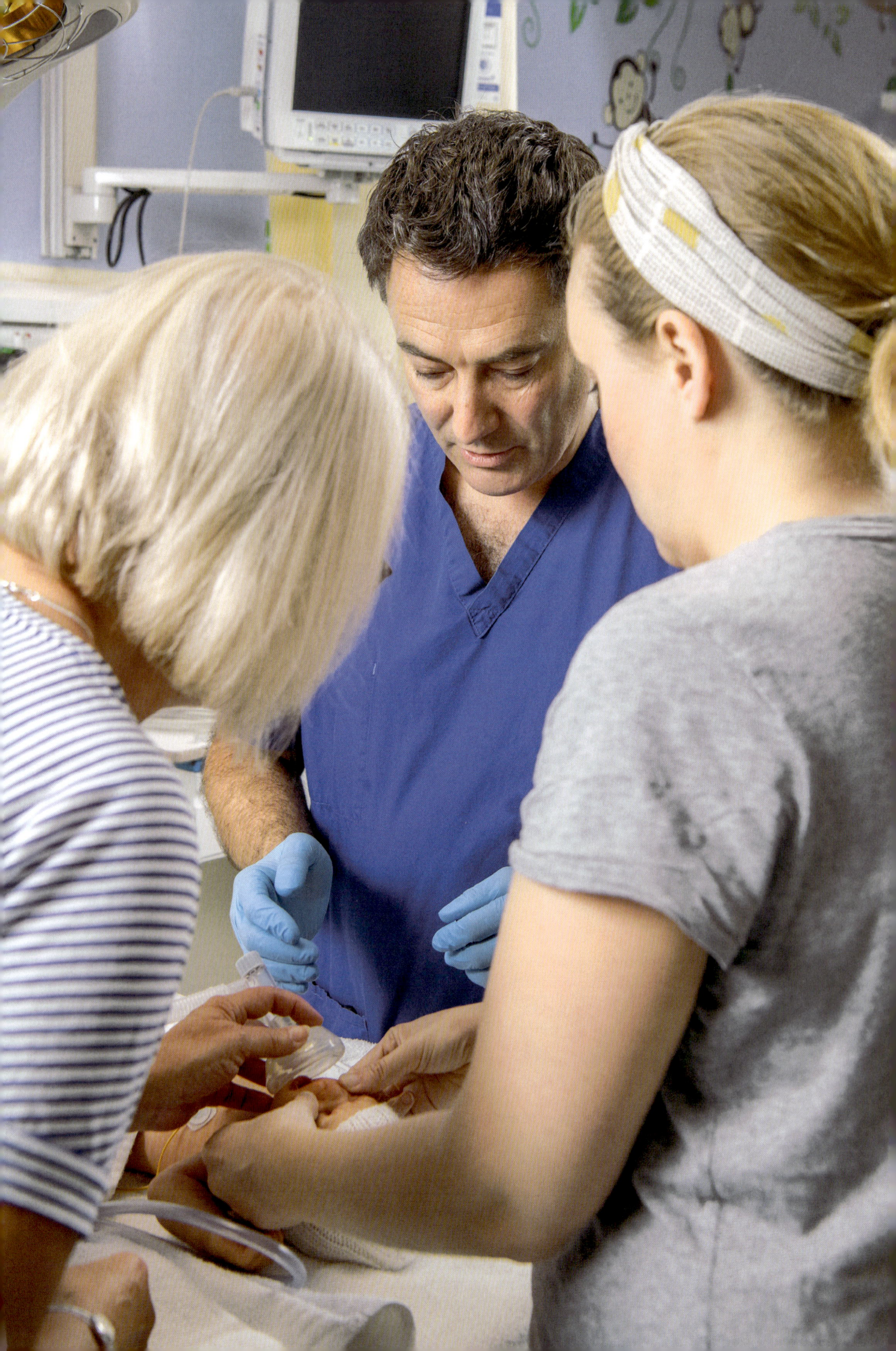

Introduction to the course

In this chapter

Aims of ARNI

The ARNI approach & algorithm

Assessment on the ARNI course

The Advanced Resuscitation of the Newborn Infant (ARNI) course has been developed, under the auspices of Resuscitation Council UK, to build on the foundations provided in the Newborn Life Support (NLS) course. This manual provides course material for the ARNI course. However, it will be a useful resource for all neonatal care providers.

The ARNI course aims to provide clear, practical instruction enabling individuals to work within a team to stabilise preterm and sick term babies. It focuses on a range of common emergencies and deals with extreme prematurity and some of the congenital problems faced when providing neonatal intensive care. This manual is not intended to be a comprehensive textbook of neonatology but rather a useful resource that should give course participants and other neonatal care providers a framework on which to base their practice.

The ARNI course has been developed for NLS providers who have ongoing involvement in neonatal care and are working in a capacity where they may be called on to be a key member of a resuscitation team or provide intensive care, however briefly, to any baby from their birth until discharge home.

Aims of ARNI

- To re-establish and build upon NLS competencies.
- To give experienced staff the knowledge and skills to stabilise infants born extremely preterm, very sick or with congenital abnormalities.
- To use the ARNI algorithm and approach to assess a newborn infant or a baby in a neonatal setting and recognise worrying and potentially life-threatening clinical features.
- To give the knowledge and skills needed to deal with common emergencies affecting infants within neonatal and maternity unit settings using a logical approach.

   A   B   C   D   E   F

- To be able to work effectively within a team to provide resuscitation or intensive care to a baby.
- To support staff in providing clear, open and sensitive communication with families.

The course concentrates on the effective teaching of practical and teamworking skills.

Learning outcomes

Having read the manual and completed an ARNI course you should:

1. Understand a structured approach to resuscitation in neonatal and maternity unit settings and the principles behind this structure including the importance of airway management and lung aeration.
2. Have been taught, practised and received feedback on management of the newborn airway including performing the following skills on manikins:
   - airway management and lung aeration with feedback on mask leak
   - visualisation of the vocal cords with a laryngoscope
   - safe approach to tracheal intubation
   - an approach to the management of the difficult airway.

3. Have undertaken workshops covering management of a pneumothorax and therapeutic hypothermia.
4. Understand the human factors that facilitate effective team working and be able to recognise that some human factors may also impair or adversely affect outcomes resulting in the team not working as effectively.
5. Have practised the immediate management of a variety of neonatal emergencies in simulations, appreciating the importance of communication and teamwork.
6. Have demonstrated a structured approach to assessing and managing preterm or sick infants, as part of a team, on labour ward and the neonatal unit.
7. Have developed the skills to effectively handover and document a baby's care.
8. Have practiced communicating with families in difficult circumstances.

The ARNI approach

The ARNI approach involves good preparation, planning and communication. This enables a rapid initial airway, breathing and circulation (ABC) assessment to be made. Each of A, B and C should be rapidly categorised as potentially life-threatening, worrying or satisfactory. Any potentially life-threatening findings need to be dealt with immediately.

Following the initial rapid ABC assessment and immediate actions a follow up ABCDEF assessment should be done:

A Airway

B Breathing

C Circulation

D Disability / drugs / dextrose

E Environment / everything else

F Family

Categorisation of levels of concern (potentially life-threatening, worrying, satisfactory) should be reassessed during the follow on ABCDEF assessment.

The rapid initial ABC assessment identifies the need for immediate cardiopulmonary resuscitation (CPR). If there are no immediate life-threatening features then further ABCDEF reassessment helps clarify management priorities, initiate stabilising treatments and work towards a definitive plan or diagnosis. This approach is shown in the ARNI algorithm (Figure 1.1).

Assessment on the ARNI Course

The ARNI course assesses technical and non-technical skills. In order to pass, the aims of the ARNI course must be met:
- be able to work effectively within a team to provide resuscitation or intensive care to a neonate
- support staff in providing clear, open and sensitive communication with families.

Assessed parts of the course are:
- Airway skills, including demonstrating:
  – safe, effective mask ventilation
  – safe practice before, during and after tracheal intubation – although successful intubation of a manikin is not required to pass the course.
- Simulations and workshops are assessed throughout the course in a formative way using continuous assessment. Feedback will be given with advice on areas for improvement.

Why is ARNI needed?

Neonatal networks try to centralise the care of extremely preterm babies to neonatal intensive care units and improved antenatal scanning predicts many congenital problems. However, there will always be unexpected deliveries or babies that need resuscitation in all centres. For this reason, the ARNI course is aimed at all staff who work with babies not just neonatal intensive care staff. A substantial amount of neonatal care is provided outside neonatal intensive care units in the UK and the ARNI approach and the skills taught on the course will be valuable to a wide range of health care professionals.

A number of national reviews from the Project 27/28 in 2005 to the RCOG Each Baby Counts and the Year 3 Maternity Incentive Scheme report from NHS Resolution in 2020 have highlighted a substantial proportion of neonatal deaths or morbidity were associated with deficiencies in the early care provided to preterm infants.

There is a national drive in the UK to reduce stillbirths, neonatal deaths and the number of babies left severely disabled as a result of incidents that occur during term labour.

Whilst survival for extremely preterm infants continues to improve; there is still significant morbidity in surviving infants. It is essential that all staff caring for sick babies are able to provide effective resuscitation and stabilisation. These are skills that need to be maintained, as early recognition of problems and appropriate intervention really do make a difference.

Advanced resuscitation of the newborn infant

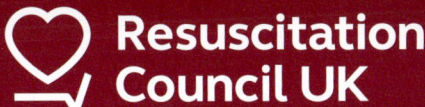

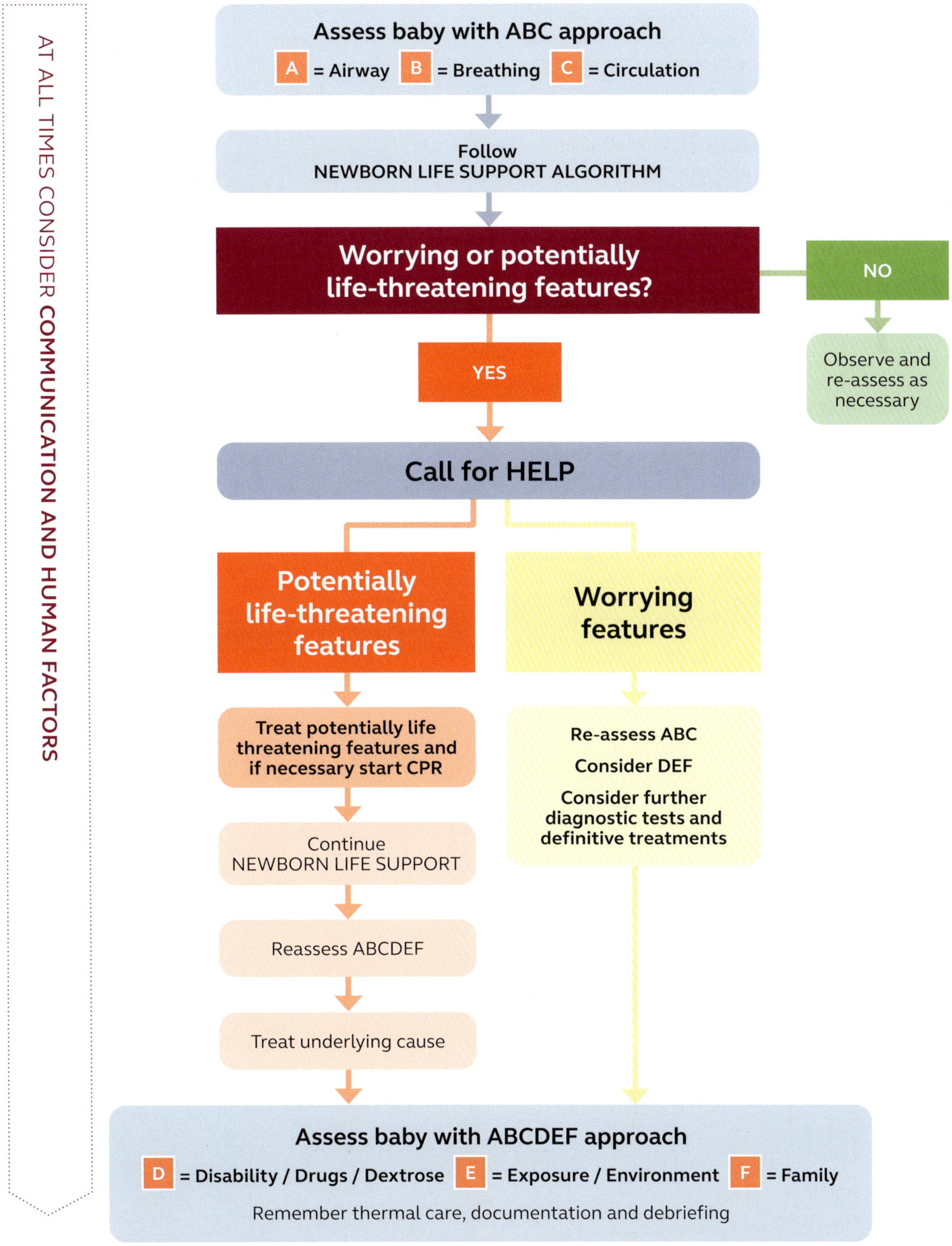

Figure 1.1 The ARNI algorithm

Science and guidelines

The International Liaison Committee on Resuscitation (ILCOR) and Emergency Cardiovascular Care Science with Treatment Recommendations (CoSTR) are the result of a continuous cycle of evidence review done in collaboration between resuscitation experts from around the world.

The resuscitation guidelines in this manual are consistent with the European Resuscitation Council guidelines and the Newborn resuscitation and support of transition of infants at birth guidelines.

Where drug doses are given these have been checked against international guidelines or relevant national formularies however readers are reminded of the need to check all drug doses carefully.

Further reading

Macintosh M, ed. CESDI. Project 27/28. An enquiry into quality of care and its effect on the survival of babies born at 27–28 weeks. London: The Stationery Office, 2003.

Newborn Life Support; Resuscitation at Birth. 5th ed. Resuscitation Council UK, London, 2021.

NHS Resolution Sept 2019. The Early Notification scheme progress report: collaboration and improved experience for families. https://resolution.nhs.uk/resources/early-notification-scheme-progress-report/

Royal College of Obstetrics and Gynaecology https://www.rcog.org.uk/eachbabycounts

Wyckoff MH, Weiner GM, et al. Neonatal Life Support 2020 International Consensus on Cardiopulmonary Resuscitation and Emergency Cardiovascular Care Science With Treatment Recommendations. Pediatrics. 2020; doi: 10.1542/peds.2020-038505C.

My key take-home messages from this chapter are:

Resuscitation at birth

02

In this chapter

The standard NLS approach to resuscitation at birth

Preparation for a baby that may require resuscitation at birth

Umbilical cord management

Assessment and reassessment of the baby

More complex resuscitation situations

Unresponsive babies and how long to continue resuscitation

The learning outcomes will enable you to:

Review the NLS approach to resuscitation at birth

Understand that basic resuscitation underpins advanced resuscitation

Be able to follow an 'ABCDEF' approach to a more complex resuscitation at birth

Introduction

The need for resuscitation at birth is often unpredictable. Anyone attending deliveries should be able to start basic resuscitation until more senior help arrives. Sometimes ARNI providers are the more senior help. The majority of babies will respond quickly to simple resuscitation manoeuvres.

There are some situations that make resuscitation at birth more challenging. Examples might include:

- extremely preterm infants (Chapter 3)
- babies born with congenital abnormalities affecting the airway; for example, cleft palate or Pierre Robin sequence (Chapter 7)
- babies born with congenital abnormities or conditions affecting the chest, for example, congenital diaphragmatic hernia, pulmonary hypoplasia or hydrops fetalis
- babies in terminal apnoea who not respond to initial resuscitation measures
- multiple births
- difficult deliveries, for example, shoulder dystocia or cord prolapse.

When facing potentially challenging resuscitation, it is important that the basic airway techniques learnt on the NLS course and the NLS algorithm (Figure 2.1) are used appropriately; these form the basis for advanced resuscitation.

A B C D E F

A rapid initial ABC assessment followed by an 'ABCDEF' reassessment provides structure, even in complicated resuscitation (see Chapter 1). Catagorisation of each area into potentially life-threatening, worrying or satisfactory helps establish important clinical priorities.

> Anyone attending deliveries should be able to start basic resuscitation until more senior help arrives

Preparation

If there is time:

- Make yourself known to the parents and explain why you are there.
- Review the maternal notes to identify any important factors that may affect the baby, including any advanced care directives that may have been agreed.
- Consider your team: if a challenging resuscitation is anticipated, call for help early.
- Wash your hands, put on gloves and if necessary PPE, prepare the resuscitation area.
- Make sure any heater is on, the environmental temperature is adequate and that doors and windows are closed.
- Ensure there are enough warm towels (plastic bags for small preterm babies).
- Check the gas supply and delivery system including a T-piece or self-inflating bag. and a range of suitable sized face masks.
- Ensure air / oxygen blender settings and pressure limits are set appropriately.
- Check that a pulse oximeter and probe are available.
- Check that the suction works and is set appropriately with the right type and size of catheter.
- Ensure that airway adjuncts are available (e.g. laryngeal mask, oropharyngeal airways and working laryngoscope).
- If intubation is anticipated, prepare an appropriately sized tracheal tube, a suitable method to secure the tube and an end tidal CO_2 detector.
- Check venous access equipment and resuscitation drugs.
- Check that the clock works.
- If preterm consider having surfactant available with a suitable delivery device.

Consider

- Do you have the staff you need for this delivery? More hands may be needed for multiple births, extreme prematurity or complex situations and the most senior support available may be required. As a team gets larger the human factors discussed in Chapter 5 become more important; for example, do the members of the team have allocated roles?
- Is transport to the neonatal unit likely to be required? If the baby is likely to be very small or preterm then arrange to have a system for transfer to the neonatal unit. Think about how you will manage the airway, breathing, monitoring and thermal control during transfer.

Anticipation can often prevent difficulties and in some situations the need for support is predictable e.g. extreme prematurity, antenatally diagnosed congenital abnormalities. It is better to have help arrive and not need it than to find you really need help which has not yet been summoned.

Do you need help? Don't be proud. Always ask for help if you expect or encounter any difficulty.

Umbilical cord management

The optimal time of cord clamping has been widely studied and delayed cord clamping (DCC) is safe and does not increase maternal adverse outcomes (e.g. postpartum haemorrhage). The terms 'delayed and 'deferred' are often used interchangeably.

The preferred cord management options are:

1. 60 s of DCC unless it would prevent immediate resuscitation measures that are felt to be necessary
2. If resuscitation is required and 60 s of DCC is not practical then cord milking (intact or cut cord) is an option in babies > 28 weeks gestation
3. Occasionally immediate cord clamping may be needed (Table 2.1)
4. Cord management requires planning and communication between the teams involved and with the parents.

Delayed cord clamping

There have been three recent meta-analyses looking at delayed cord clamping with slightly different studies included in each meta-analysis. Whilst the degree of benefit reported varies, they consistently report that the main neonatal benefit is reduced mortality in preterm infants. The most recent ILCOR systematic review reports one extra survivor for every 50 babies who received DCC. The benefit is greater in babies < 30 weeks with one extra survivor for every 33 babies who received DCC.

Additional neonatal benefits include avoiding immediate cord clamping induced bradycardia, less labile arterial blood pressure and a more physiological transition. Benefits over the first 24 h are higher haemoglobin, higher mean BP and less use of inotropes. Later benefits are a higher haematocrit at 7 days and fewer blood transfusions.

There is no universally accepted definition of DCC, only that it does not occur immediately after the infant is born. Recent systematic reviews and meta-analyses have considered delayed cord clamping as being clamping at a time longer than 30 s after birth. Other studies suggest that longer clamping times may be beneficial as long as the baby can be kept warm. A different approach has

Resuscitation Council UK
GUIDELINES 2021

Newborn life support

(Antenatal counselling)
Team briefing and equipment check

Birth
Delay cord clamping if possible

Start clock / note time
Dry / wrap, stimulate, keep warm

Assess
Colour, tone, breathing, heart rate

Ensure an open airway
Preterm: consider CPAP

If gasping / not breathing
- Give 5 inflations (30 cm H_2O) – start in air
- Apply PEEP 5–6 cm H_2O, if possible
- Apply SpO_2 +/- ECG

Reassess
If no increase in heart rate, look for chest movement

If the chest is not moving
- Check mask, head and jaw position
- 2 person support
- Consider suction, laryngeal mask/tracheal tube
- Repeat inflation breaths
- Consider increasing the inflation pressure

Reassess
If no increase in heart rate, look for chest movement

Once chest is moving continue ventilation breaths

If heart rate is not detectable or < 60 min^{-1} after 30 seconds of ventilation
- Synchronise 3 chest compressions to 1 ventilation
- Increase oxygen to 100%
- Consider intubation if not already done or laryngeal mask if not possible

Reassess heart rate and chest movement every 30 seconds

If the heart rate remains not detectable or < 60 min^{-1}
- **Vascular access and drugs**
- Consider other factors e.g. pneumothorax, hypovolaemia, congenital abormality

Update parents and debrief team
Complete records

Preterm < 32 weeks

Place undried in plastic wrap + radiant heat

Inspired oxygen
28–31 weeks 21–30%
< 28 weeks 30%

If giving inflations, start with 25 cm H_2O

Acceptable pre-ductal SpO_2	
2 min	65%
5 min	85%
10 min	90%

TITRATE OXYGEN TO ACHIEVE TARGET SATURATIONS

APPROX 60 SECONDS

MAINTAIN TEMPERATURE

AT ALL TIMES ASK "IS HELP NEEDED"

Figure 2.1   Newborn life support algorithm

been to consider physiological changes e.g. delaying cord clamping until after the lungs have been aerated.

RCUK recommends that, if possible, the umbilical cord should not be clamped until at least 60 s after birth. Additionally, ILCOR, the European Resuscitation Council and the World Health Organisation have similar recommendations. Achieving this as part of the stabilisation process requires planning and should feature in the pre-delivery team brief.

DCC for healthy babies

In the healthy baby, 60 s of DCC can simply occur whilst the baby is being dried and gently stimulated; the baby is then placed skin-to-skin on the mother's abdomen and covered to ensure they remain warm. Assessment of the baby's colour, tone, breathing and heart rate can be undertaken during this period which will probably take about 30 s. The baby who is crying needs no further support, but close observation, and possible intervention, is needed if they do not cry.

DCC for the baby that does not cry at birth

If the baby is not crying, they should be closely assessed. Some parts of the standard algorithm, for example, opening the airway, can be undertaken whilst the baby remains skin-to-skin. If additional support is needed then a resuscitaire is usually required. The team must then make a choice whether to clamp the cord and take the baby to the resuscitaire, or whether to leave the cord unclamped and to bring a resuscitaire or other bedside stabilisation device to the baby. Local policy and facilities will probably dictate which route is followed.

DCC for babies that require resuscitation

Optimal umbilical cord management in babies that require resuscitation is subject to ongoing research. At present there is insufficient evidence to make a recommendation about DCC when resuscitation is required.

With appropriate preparation and training resuscitation whilst undertaking DCC can be carried out using a standard resuscitaire or a specifically designed platform. However, the priority is to provide resuscitation that follows standard NLS and ARNI approaches. If that cannot be done effectively with the umbilical cord intact then the cord should be clamped immediately and the baby moved to a suitable resuscitation area.

Situations where DCC should not be done

There are a number of situations when DCC may not be possible or may not be wanted (Table 2.1).

Table 2.1 Situations where cord clamping may not be possible or may not be helpful

Not possible	1. Cases with interruption of the placental blood flow/oxygenation: – Maternal haemorrhage – Maternal seizure or cardiac arrest – Placenta abruption – Vasa praevia – Cord avulsion
Potentially unhelpful	2. Fetal hydrops due to any underlying cause
	3. Recipient twin in placental sharing (monochorionic) twins

Umbilical cord milking

When DCC is not possible, alternatives in babies > 28 weeks gestation include intact cord milking and cut cord milking which both offer advantages for the baby over immediate umbilical cord clamping.

There are two types of cord milking:

1. Umbilical cord milking with an intact cord: the umbilical cord is gently grasped as far away from the baby as possible, and milked towards the baby, usually 3–5 times. This can result in a faster blood flow than occurs with passive blood return due to uterine contraction. During the milkings, a term infant may receive about 50 mL of blood. After milking the cord is clamped and cut and the baby is taken to the resuscitaire.

2. Umbilical cord milking from a length of cut cord: In this procedure the cord is clamped as far away from the baby as possible. In a term baby this gives about 25 cm of cord (less in a preterm baby where cords are usually shorter). The baby is taken to the resuscitaire immediately and milking is undertaken in a similar manner to that described above.

An International Liaison Committee on Resuscitation (ILCOR) and Cochrane meta-analysis of DCC, intact and cut cord milking strategies showed that all three had similar benefits. However, DCC was the preferred method of providing placental transfusion as this was the more physiological option.

Umbilical cord milking safety

Cord milking is not recommended in infants < 28 weeks' gestation.

Although, compared with DCC, intact cord milking appeared to offer similar benefits, one large study of intact cord milking versus DCC was terminated early when analysis demonstrated a significant excess of severe intraventricular haemorrhage in infants born before 28 weeks in the cord milking group.

Furthermore, animal studies of cord milking demonstrate marked haemodynamic fluctuations in arterial blood pressure and cerebral blood flow which are thought to be potentially injurious to the immature cerebral circulation.

After delivery

1. Start the clock or note the time of birth.
2. Umbilical cord management.
3. Assess the baby whilst considering thermal care (see below).
4. For a term baby, dry the baby quickly and effectively. Remove the wet towel and wrap in a fresh dry warm towel. Very small or significantly preterm babies should be placed into a clear plastic bag or wrap without drying and a radiant heater should be used.
5. Assess the heart rate, breathing, tone and colour.
6. Clamp and cut the cord.

Stimulation

The stress of delivery will stimulate the baby, as will the subsequent handling and drying. This is usually sufficient.

Initial assessment

- Colour
- Tone
- Breathing
- Heart Rate

Heart rate

In healthy term babies who received immediate cord clamping, the median (IQR) HR was 96 (65–127) beats per min (bpm) at 1 min, rising at 2 min to 139 (110–166) bpm and 5 min to 163 (146–175) bpm respectively. Babies who received delayed cord clamping do not experience an immediate cord clamping induced bradycardia and have a higher HR at a minute of age. Heart rate rises more slowly in preterm babies and those born by caesarean section. Adequate lung inflation will usually lead to a rapid rise in heart rate as long as the heart is pumping enough to move oxygenated blood the short distance from the lungs to the heart.

When first assessing the heart rate, use a stethoscope. It is usually straightforward to categorise the heart rate as very slow (less than 60 bpm), slow (60–100 bpm) or fast (more than 100 bpm). It is not necessary to count the heart rate with complete accuracy. Heart rate assessment by stethoscope is more accurate than by palpating cord pulsation at the base of the umbilicus which may not reflect the true heart rate.

Breathing

Breathing usually starts spontaneously within a minute of birth and whilst apnoea on assessment may warrant action, it is important to realise that some perfectly healthy babies can take up to three minutes to start breathing after birth. The baby may show normal regular breaths, irregular breaths, gasping (sometimes interspersed amongst more normal breaths), or breathing may be absent (apnoea).

Gasping breaths are usually accompanied by recession, but recession is also occasionally seen with regular breathing, suggesting increased work of breathing. This may be due to partial obstruction of the airway or lung disease in premature babies.

If the baby is mature, has a good heart rate and is making good respiratory effort then no further help is required. Once wrapped, this baby should be given to the parents.

Tone

Babies born well-flexed and with good tone are usually healthy. A term baby who is very floppy is likely to be in significant difficulty. The tone of a baby is often clear from its posture but can also be rapidly assessed when handling the baby. Preterm babies commonly have reduced tone compared to term babies.

Colour

After the initial assessment, colour does not appear in the NLS algorithm because it is not a good way of assessing oxygenation or whether oxygenation is improving However, it is mentioned here because it is still thought to be useful for assessing the initial condition of the baby at birth.

A baby in difficulty resulting from acidosis or significant blood loss will appear very pale. A well baby will often appear blue at birth but will become pink over the first few minutes of life. Very pale babies who remain pale after resuscitation may be hypovolaemic as well as acidotic.

Pulse oximetry

Using a pulse oximeter will allow accurate assessment of heart rate and oxygen saturation within about 60–90 s of application. A stethoscope is the most reliable means of monitoring heart rate until the pulse oximeter picks up a reliable trace. Saturation levels in healthy babies in the first few minutes of life may be considerably lower than at other times (Table 2.2). In babies at birth the

Table 2.2 Acceptable pre-ductal saturations over the first 10 min of life

Time from birth	Acceptable pre-ductal saturations
2 min	65%
5 min	85%
10 min	90%

arterial oxygen saturation may be different depending on whether it is measured in areas supplied by blood leaving the aorta before or after the entry of the arterial duct; i.e. whether they are pre-ductal or post-ductal measurements. Measurements taken in the right arm are pre-ductal whereas measurements from other limbs will be post-ductal. Pre-ductal saturations reflect cerebral oxygenation levels.

Pre-ductal oxygen saturation values in the Table 2.2 are taken from babies of all gestations in a study of over 450 healthy babies who received no resuscitation and no additional oxygen in the minutes immediately after birth. The data came from 308 term babies, 121 babies between 32 and 36 weeks gestation and 39 babies under 32 weeks gestation.

The saturation levels listed in this table are deemed 'acceptable' in the sense that babies exhibiting these levels probably do not need any supplemental oxygen. Resuscitation of term infants should commence in air. For preterm infants, < 28 weeks 30% oxygen should be used, for those 28–32 weeks 21–30%. If, despite effective ventilation, oxygenation (ideally guided by oximetry) remains unacceptable, use of a higher concentration of oxygen should be considered. Blended oxygen and air should be given judiciously and its use guided by pulse oximetry. If a blend of oxygen and air is not available, use what is available. If chest compressions are administered, supplemental oxygen should be increased to 100%. Babies with oxygen saturations of 95% or more do not need supplemental oxygen.

ECG estimation of heart rate

An ECG can give a rapid, accurate and continuous assessment of heart rate reading during newborn resuscitation. It does not, however, indicate the presence of a cardiac output and should not be the sole means of monitoring the infant. The leads should be applied to the body as they do not stay well attached to the limbs. Care should be taken to minimise skin trauma when applying adhesive leads to extremely preterm infants.

Airway opening manoeuvres

If a baby is not breathing adequately, or is gasping, then the first step is to open the airway. The airway may be obstructed if the neck is either too flexed or too extended. If a baby with low tone is placed on its back there may be airway obstruction due to lack of oropharyngeal tone. These mechanisms are more likely to be the cause of an airway problem than any mechanical obstruction from blood, thick mucus, or lumps of vernix or meconium.

If a congenital abnormality of the airway is suspected, an airway adjunct (laryngeal mask, oropharyngeal or nasopharyngeal airway) can be very useful.

After opening the airway and giving stimulation some babies start to make satisfactory breathing efforts, in which case the airway should continue to be supported and the baby observed. Reassess the heart rate to ensure this is satisfactory.

Meconium

Routine suctioning for infants born through meconium stained liquor is not recommended and the standard NLS approach should be followed for these babies. The emphasis should be on initiating lung inflation within the first minute of life in non-breathing or ineffectively breathing infants and this should not be delayed. Tracheal intubation is not routinely required in the presence of meconium but is an important option if tracheal obstruction is suspected.

Screaming babies	Have an open airway
Floppy babies	Start routine NLS algorithm
	If chest rise is not obtained, inspect under direct vision and suction if necessary.
	Focus on aerating the lungs in a timely manner.

Inflation breaths

In order to clear lung fluid in an unresponsive newborn baby, positive pressure inflations lasting 2–3 s are required. For a term baby, start at pressures of 30 cm water. Five such 'inflation breaths' should be sufficient to aerate the lung if the airway is open. Significantly preterm babies (32 weeks and below) may well respond to a lower initial inflation pressure of 25 cm water. In all babies > 32 weeks start resuscitation with air, in babies 28–32 weeks start in 21–30% oxygen, babies < 28 weeks should start in 30%. Supplemental oxygen may be used if the saturation levels remain below the expected level.

Positive end expiratory pressure (PEEP) has been shown to be helpful in resuscitation at birth in babies of all gestations. A PEEP of 5 cm water would be a commonly used initial setting.

Following 5 inflation breaths – reassess to see if the baby has responded.

Reassess – has the heart rate improved?

Heart rate is increasing

If inflation breaths have aerated the lung you would expect the heart rate to increase within 5–10 s. This is one of the first signs that the baby is responding. If the heart rate is increasing rapidly then you can assume that you have successfully aerated the lungs. You then proceed as follows:

Ventilation support
Following inflation breaths, the baby may start breathing spontaneously. If this does not occur, gently ventilate the lungs at about 30 breaths min^{-1} until the baby starts to breathe. If ventilation is adequate the heart rate will remain above 100 bpm. If it falls below

Table 2.3 Neonatal resuscitation drug doses

Drug	Dose	Route	
Adrenaline (epinephrine)	0.2 mL kg^{-1} of 1:10 000 (20 micrograms kg^{-1}) (for first and subsequent doses)	UVC, IV or IO	To stimulate the heart. Repeat every 3–5 min if CPR is ongoing.
	1 mL kg^{-1} 1:10 000 (100 microgram kg^{-1})	Tracheal tube	Only give tracheal adrenaline, whilst trying to gain UVC/IO access
Dextrose	2.5 mL kg^{-1} of 10%	UVC, IV or IO	As the heart cannot work without glucose and many babies will have depleted their cardiac glycogen stores by this stage of a resuscitation
Volume	10 mL kg^{-1} 0.9% sodium chloride (rarely O negative blood required for acute blood loss)	UVC, IV or IO	
Sodium Bicarbonate	1–2 mmol kg^{-1} (2–4 mL kg^{-1} of 4.2% sodium bicarbonate) or (1–2 mL kg^{-1} of 8.4% sodium bicarbonate diluted 1:1 with water or 5% dextrose)	UVC, IV or IO	To improve intracellular acidosis thus making the myocardium more responsive to adrenaline

this it suggests that ventilation is inadequate in some way. Recheck the airway position and mask seal. Pressures of around 25 cm water and inspiratory times of 1 s or less are usually adequate for ventilation once the initial lung fluid has been displaced. Certain situations may require less pressure (hypoxic ischaemic encephalopathy without meconium aspiration) or more pressure (pulmonary hypoplasia). Adequate pressure delivery can be assessed in the first instance by achieving an adequate heart rate and secondly by observing the degree of chest wall movement.

Reassess – is there spontaneous breathing?
With continued support, breathing efforts will usually return. The manner in which these return is important. If the first efforts are gasping in nature, this would suggest that the baby may have been in terminal apnoea. It is important to record the sequence and timing of events. If the heart rate is satisfactory but no spontaneous breathing returns then you might consider other factors such as sedation, neurological issues or intrathoracic pathology. Remember, it is possible to decrease a baby's respiratory drive by inadvertently lowering the pCO$_2$ with hyperventilation.

Heart rate is not increasing

If the heart rate is not responding, the most likely reason is that the lungs have not been inflated. Under these circumstances, go back and check the airway and mask position and repeat the inflation breaths. Consider using airway support and/or other airway manoeuvres such as a two-person jaw thrust, laryngeal mask or an oropharyngeal airway.

Reassess – is there chest movement?
In the absence of a heart rate response, seeing the chest move as you give inflation breaths is the only way to judge successful aeration of the lungs. Listening for breath sounds with a stethoscope can be misleading because of transmitted upper airway sounds. Chest movement may only start to occur after the first few (two or three) effective inflation breaths. Check for chest movement with further inflation breaths. Once chest rise is confirmed, if the heart rate is < 100, 30 s of ventilation breaths should be given.

Reassess – is the heart rate satisfactory?
If the heart rate remains slow or absent, despite 30 s of adequate ventilation as shown by chest movement, then the supplemental oxygen should be increased to 100% and chest compressions started. Chest compressions help to move oxygenated blood from the lungs to the heart and coronary arteries. The blood you move can only be oxygenated if the lungs have been successfully aerated.

The recommended compression: ventilation ratio for CPR is 3:1 for newborn resuscitation. Asynchronous chest compressions are not recommended in newborn resuscitation, even if the baby is intubated.

If you have the skills, tracheal intubation should be considered to help maintain the airway. If intubation skills are not available, use of a laryngeal mask can help secure the airway. Correct tracheal tube placement should be confirmed by auscultation and detection of exhaled carbon dioxide with colour change capnography (Chapter 7). Remember that colour change capnography is unreliable in babies with poor cardiac output.

Reassess – has the heart rate improved?
It is usually only necessary to continue chest compressions for about 20–30 s before the heart responds with an increase in heart rate.

Consider drugs
If the baby has been subjected to severe hypoxic stress then adequate ventilation and chest compressions may not be enough to produce an increase in heart rate. In this situation it may be necessary to use drugs. The drugs commonly used in neonatal resuscitation are ourlined in Table 2.3.

The venous access necessary to give these drugs is most easily achieved using an umbilical venous catheter (UVC). A less commonly used option is intraosseous (IO) access. A less effective option is administration via a tracheal tube; however, this route can only be used for adrenaline.

Reassess – has the heart rate improved?
If the heart rate is still not improving consider other factors such as hypovolaemia, tension pneumothorax, diaphragmatic hernia or, rarely, complete heart block.

Reassess – should resuscitation attempts continue?
If there was no detectable heart rate at birth and still none by 10–20 min of age, survival is unlikely and long-term serious neurological disability amongst survivors is very likely. It is entirely appropriate to consider stopping resuscitation after discussion with a senior member of the team and involving the family.

If the heart rate remains slow at 10–20 min and is not improving the outlook is still very poor but the situation is more complex and senior advice should be urgently sought if not already done so.

More complex resuscitation situations

Some situations can make resuscitation more complex and many of these are covered throughout the ARNI manual and course. Examples are:
- Extremely preterm infants (Chapter 3)
- Congenital airway abnormalities (Chapter 7)
- Congenital diaphragmatic hernia (Chapter 9)
- Pulmonary hypoplasia
- Hydrops fetalis.

Babies who do not respond to initial resuscitation measures

These are the babies that are likely to require most of the interventions described in the NLS algorithm including cardiac compressions and potentially drugs. The most senior staff available should be called to assist and a full resuscitation team is likely to be needed. Issues that may arise are:
- Need for urgent IV access via an emergency UVC, if that is not possible an IO could be considered.
- If there is a history of antepartum haemorrhage, abruption or cord rupture, whether emergency O negative blood transfusion is required. With extreme blood loss, the heart rate may not rise above 100 bpm until the circulation is supported.
- After a baby has been resuscitated whether therapeutic hypothermia is indicated. Remember to complete the ABC of resuscitation before commencing either passive or active cooling.
- Regardless of outcome clear discussions with traumatised parents about the situation will need to occur involving senior staff. Communication with families is discussed further in Chapter 6.

Multiple births present the logistical problem of having to deal with more than one baby at once. Careful planning is needed to ensure that adequate members of appropriately trained staff are available to assist.

When to stop resuscitation

The previous 2015 recommendations of discontinuing resuscitation have been reconsidered as it can take longer than 10 min to complete all the steps of the NLS algorithm. Additionally, small numbers of survivors occasionally without moderate to severe neurodevelopmental impairment, have been reported after resuscitation lasting over 10 min. This prompted an ILCOR systematic review to consider the evidence around prolonged resuscitation of newborn infants. Although the available evidence is of very low certainty, they were able to make the following comments and give a weak recommendation.

"Failure to achieve return of spontaneous circulation in newborn infants despite 10 to 20 min of intensive resuscitation is associated with a high risk of mortality and a high risk of moderate-to-severe neurodevelopmental impairment among survivors.

However, there is no evidence that any specific duration of resuscitation consistently predicts mortality or moderate-to-severe neurodevelopmental impairment. If, despite provision of all the recommended steps of resuscitation and excluding reversible causes, a newborn infant requires on-going cardiopulmonary resuscitation (CPR) after birth, we suggest discussion of discontinuing resuscitative efforts with the clinical team and family. A reasonable time frame to consider this change in goals of care is around 20 min after birth."

The difficulty of this decision-making emphasises the need for senior help to be sought as soon as possible.

Transferring to the neonatal unit (NNU)

The NNU should be alerted as soon as practical, so that they can prepare a cot space with appropriate equipment to provide ongoing care. Transfer from the delivery area to NNU should be planned to minimise the destabilising effect of transfer, and with the ability to deal with any clinical deterioration that may occur whilst moving the baby. The SBAR approach (Chapter 5) can be helpful to use during handover to the neonatal unit team.

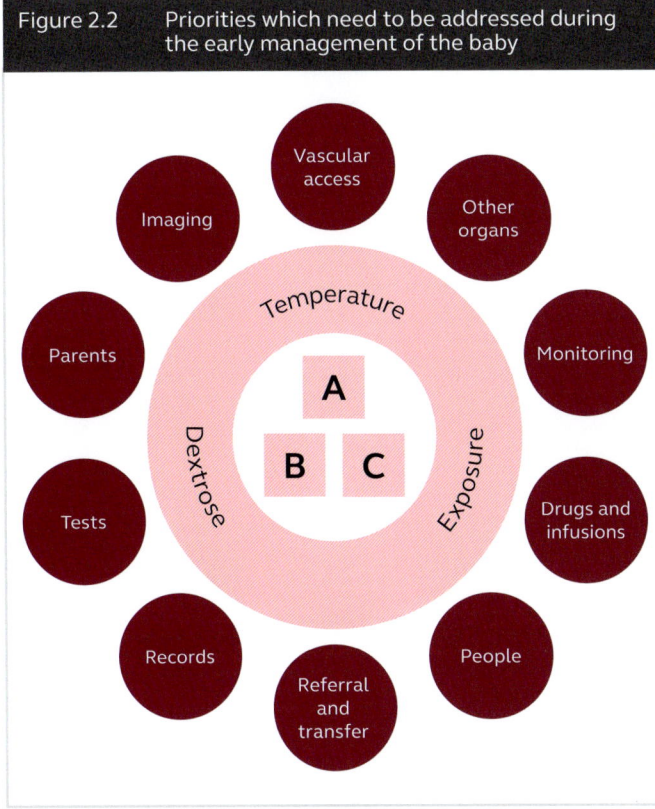

Figure 2.2 Priorities which need to be addressed during the early management of the baby

Early postnatal management priorities

A number of assessments and actions need to be carried out once a baby is admitted to a neonatal unit. All babies require an ABCDEF reassessment on admission to the neonatal unit. Figure 2.2 indicates the range of assessments, considerations and actions that may need to occur. Use of the ARNI algorithm and approach to categorising the components of an ABCDEF assessment as satisfactory, worrying or life-threatening can clarify important priorities.

Ongoing actions are usually adjusting respiratory support as necessary, cardiorespiratory monitoring, intravenous access, antibiotic administration and updating parents.

The management of extremely premature babies is considered in Chapter 3.

In unstable babies' early recognition of problems and intervention to prevent deterioration is very important, this is covered in more detail in Chapter 4.

02: Summary learning

Follow the NLS algorithm
- If possible, brief team and anticipate problems
- Consider thermal control (i.e. remove the wet towel, dry and cover baby)
- Airway
- Breathing – inflation breaths, followed by ventilation breaths
- Chest compressions
- (Drugs)

If a baby Is not responding to resuscitation measures consider the potential reasons why.

In a newborn baby requiring ongoing CPR after 10–20 min of resuscitation it is reasonable to consider reorientating to palliative care at around 20 min after birth.

For babies being admitted to the neonatal unit, the unit needs to be notified and transfer from labour ward to the unit needs to carefully planned.

My key take-home messages from this chapter are:

Further reading

BAPM Optimal Cord Management in Preterm Babies A Quality Improvement Toolkit. December 2020 https://hubble-live-assets.s3.amazonaws.com/bapm/redactor2_assets/files/814/OCM_Toolkit_Full_For_Launch.pdf

Dawson J, Kamlin C, Wong C et al. Changes in heart rate in the first minutes after birth. Arch Dis Child Fetal Neonatal Ed 2010; 95: F177-F181.

Chettri S, Adhisivam B, Bhat BV. Endotracheal suction for nonvigorous neonates born through meconium stained amniotic fluid: a randomized controlled trial. J Pediatr 2015; 166: 1208-13.e1.

Dawson JA, Kamlin COF, Vento M, et al. Defining the reference range for oxygen saturation for infants after birth. Pediatrics. 2010; 125: e1340-7.

Fogarty M, Osborn DA, Askie L, Seidler AL, et al. Delayed vs early umbilical cord clamping for preterm infants: a systematic review and meta-analysis. Am J Obstet Gynecol. 2018 Jan;218(1):1-18. doi: 10.1016/j.ajog.2017.10.231. Epub 2017 Oct 30. PMID: 29097178.

Katheria A, Rich W, Finer N. Electrocardiogram provides a continuous heart rate faster than oximetry during neonatal resuscitation. Pediatrics 2012; 130: e1177-81.

Laptook AR, Salhab W, Bhaskar B; Neonatal Research Network. Admission temperature of low birth weight infants: predictors and associated morbidities. Pediatrics 2007; 119:e643-9.

Mizumoto H, Tomotaki S, Shibata H, et al. Electrocardiogram shows reliable heart rates much earlier than pulse oximetry during neonatal resuscitation. Pediatr Int 2012; 54: 205-7.

O'Donnell CPF, Kamlin COF, Davis PG, et al. Clinical assessment of infant colour at delivery. Arch Dis Child Fetal Neonatal Ed 2007; 92: F465-7.

Owen CJ, Wyllie JP. Determination of heart rate in babies at birth. Resuscitation 2004; 60: 213-7.

Rabe H, Gyte GM, Díaz-Rossello JL, Duley L. Effect of timing of umbilical cord clamping and other strategies to influence placental transfusion at preterm birth on maternal and infant outcomes. Cochrane Database Syst Rev. 2019 Sep 17;9(9):CD003248. doi: 10.1002/14651858.CD003248.pub4. PMID: 31529790; PMCID: PMC6748404.

Seidler AL, Gyte G, Rabe H, et al. Umbilical Cord Management for Newborns < 34 week's gestation: a meta-analysis. Pediatrics (in press, accepted 25 Aug 2020).

Schmolzer GM, Kamlin COF, Dawson JA. et al. Respiratory monitoring of neonatal resuscitation. Arch Dis Child Fetal Neonatal Ed 201 0; 95: F295-303.

Stenson B. Resuscitation of extremely preterm infants: The influence of positive pressure, surfactant replacement and supplemental oxygen on outcome. In: Hansen TN, McIntosh N. (eds). Current Topics in Neonatology. No 4. WB Saunders, London, 2000. pp. 125-48.

Te Pas AB, Walther FJ. A randomized, controlled trial of delivery-room respiratory management in very preterm infants. Pediatrics 2007; 120: 322-9.

Vyas H, Milner AD, Hopkin IE, Boon AW. Physiologic responses to prolonged and slow rise inflation in the resuscitation of the asphyxiated newborn infant. J Pediatr 1981; 99: 635-9.

WHO Guideline: Delayed Umbilical Cord Clamping for Improved Maternal and Infant Health and Nutrition Outcomes Geneva: World Health Organization. Copyright © World Health Organization 2014.

Wyckoff MH, Weiner GM, et al. Neonatal Life Support 2020 International Consensus on Cardiopulmonary Resuscitation and Emergency Cardiovascular Care Science With Treatment Recommendations. Pediatrics. 2020; doi: 10.1542/peds.2020-038505C.

Wyllie JP, Wyckoff MH, de Almeida MF et al. Systematic Review: NLS Family Presence During Resus Neonatal CoSTR. International Liaison Committee on Resuscitation (ILCOR) Neonatal Life Support Task Force, Nov 2020. https://costr.ilcor.org/document/systematic-review-nls-family-presence-during-resus-neonatal-costr

Management of extreme prematurity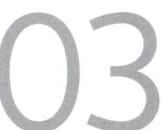

In this chapter

Important antenatal treatments that affect prognosis

Antenatal counselling

Preparation for extremely preterm delivery

Management of extremely preterm birth

Early care of the extremely preterm infant

The learning outcomes will enable you to have:

Knowledge of important antenatal treatments including steroids, magnesium sulphate and antibiotics

An awareness of factors that affect antenatal counselling

An understanding of how to stabilise the extremely preterm infant

An appreciation of when to give surfactant and options for how to administer it

An overview of invasive and non-invasive respiratory support options

An overview of early management priorities on the neonatal unit

An awareness of how early progress affects prognosis

Introduction

Infants born < 28 weeks are defined as extremely preterm and this chapter focuses on their management. It considers aspects of antenatal care and counselling, preparation and planning for extremely preterm birth, stabilisation at birth and early clinical care relevant to extreme prematurity.

Antenatal care

Although obstetric and midwifery care precedes the involvement of ARNI providers some knowledge of important antenatal treatments is useful:

Prenatal corticosteroid

A single course given to mothers with anticipated preterm delivery improves survival, reduces respiratory distress syndrome (RDS), necrotising enterocolitis (NEC) and intraventricular haemorrhage and is not associated with any significant maternal or short-term fetal adverse effects. The optimal treatment to delivery interval is > 24 h and < 7 days after the start of steroid treatment. Beneficial effects of the first dose of antenatal steroid start within a few hours. Beyond 14 days the benefits of prenatal steroid are diminished. The value of repeat doses of prenatal steroids is uncertain but both the European consensus guidelines on the management of respiratory distress syndrome (RDS) and the World Health Organisation (WHO) recommend a single repeat course of steroids. They suggest giving this 1–2 weeks after the previous course if delivery < 32 weeks is likely (European guidance) or > 7 days after the previous course if preterm birth is likely (WHO).

Magnesium sulphate

Given to women with imminent preterm delivery reduces cerebral palsy at 2 years of age by about 30% and reduces the rates of substantial motor dysfunction by about 40%. There is no significant effect on mortality. Minor maternal side effects can occur but there are no significant effects on major maternal complications.

Antenatal antibiotic use

In the context of preterm rupture of membranes maternal antibiotic use is associated with prolongation of pregnancy and improvements in a number of short-term neonatal morbidities, but no significant reduction in perinatal mortality. Markers of neonatal morbidity that are reduced are neonatal infection (RR 0.67, 95% CI 0.52 to 0.85), use of surfactant (RR 0.83, 95% CI 0.72 to 0.96) and receipt of oxygen therapy (RR 0.88, 95% CI 0.81 to 0.96). Longer term benefits are unclear with one large trial showing no difference in children's health at 7 years. Women who go into labour before 37 completed weeks of pregnancy should receive antibiotics to prevent possible transmission of group B Streptococcus. The optimal choice of antibiotic is unclear but co-amoxiclav should be avoided because of an association with necrotising enterocolitis.

Antenatal counselling

Whenever possible, parents should have the opportunity to discuss the imminent preterm birth of their baby. Antenatal counselling should:

- be influenced by information about the current gestation, estimated fetal weight, receipt of antenatal steroids and magnesium sulphate, any preterm prolonged rupture of membranes / sepsis risk factors
- consider the best estimate of current fetal wellbeing
- consider the location of birth and the level of onsite neonatal care available
- consider delivery in a centre with a tertiary neonatal intensive care unit as this is associated with increased survival
- include a reasonable overview of the possible outcomes and be informed by relevant national data and guidance
- include discussion about survival focused or comfort focused care for babies at high or extremely high risk of dying or surviving with unacceptably severe impairment
- consider parental hopes, expectations and wishes about offering resuscitation or stabilisation for the smallest and least mature babies.

The 2019 BAPM Framework on Perinatal Management of Extreme Preterm Birth before 27 weeks of gestation offers advice on risk factors that affect the chances of survival or severe disability. They consider three levels of risk of death or unacceptably severe impairment, those being extremely high (> 90%), high (> 50%) or medium (< 50%). Management orientated towards comfort focused or palliative care would usually be offered to those in the extremely high-risk category whilst those at medium-risk would usually receive survival focused care. It can be harder to know the optimal approach towards babies in the high-risk category and shared plans should be made with the family about whether resuscitation measures should be offered.

The 2019 BAPM framework estimates the prevalence of severe impairment based on 4 major studies as:

22+0 – 22+6 weeks	1-in-3 survivors
23+0 – 23+6 weeks	1-in-4 survivors
24+0 – 25+6 weeks	1-in-7 survivors
26+0 and over	1-in-10 survivors

However, families may be interested in the spectrum of developmental outcomes including rates of moderate disability, which in the EPICure 2 study were roughly comparable to the rates of severe disability in babies < 26 weeks gestation.

The condition of the baby at birth may not always correlate with survival or neurodevelopmental outcomes. However, prolonged resuscitation in the smallest and least mature babies has an extremely high risk of death or unacceptable severe disability. Consequently, the appropriateness of prolonged resuscitation including the use of resuscitation drugs needs to be very carefully considered.

Preparation and planning

Optimal management of extremely preterm infants requires skilled staff, careful coordination and correct equipment. The key preparation and planning topics covered in Chapter 2 (Figure 2.2) are all still relevant for extremely preterm infants. The topics covered in Chapter 5 are especially relevant as communication, team working, situational awareness and management of important human factors are vital to managing such small babies. Team briefing before and debriefing after delivery are important.

Dealing with the extremely preterm baby at birth

Cord management for extremely preterm infants

For uncompromised term and preterm infants, a delay in cord clamping for at least one minute from the complete delivery of the infant, is recommended.

Three meta-analyses have shown that the survival benefits of delayed cord clamping are greater in preterm babies. An ILCOR systematic review showed greater survival benefits at < 30 weeks compared to all gestations (number needed to treat 33 for < 30 weeks vs 50 for all gestations). Other metanalysis, summarised in the 2020 BAPM optimal cord management in preterm babies toolkit, reported progressively greater reductions in mortality at < 32 weeks and < 28 weeks.

Umbilical cord milking from an intact or cut cord is not recommended for preterm infants < 28 weeks due to concerns over an increase in IVH secondary to increased cerebral blood flow. Further information about cord management is provided in Chapter 2.

The concept of 'assisted transition'

Preterm babies are fragile and usually in need of assisted transition to postnatal life rather than aggressive resuscitation. Gentle intervention and minimal handling are important.

Where resuscitative measures are required and cannot be undertaken with the cord intact then resuscitation remains a priority. Stabilisation or resuscitation should follow the standard NLS approach. Factors to consider that are especially relevant to extremely preterm infants are shown in Table 3.1.

Table 3.1 Factors to consider that are especially relevant to extremely preterm infants

	Thermal care	Extremely preterm babies get cold very quickly and their mortality increases by 28% for each degree drop below 36.5°C. An overhead heater, plastic bag should be used and possibly a chemical warming mattress under a sheet. Temperature monitoring is important.
A	Airway	Be aware that airway adjuncts may be too large for the smallest babies. Gentle use of suction/ laryngoscope, if needed, to avoid soft tissue damage. If intubating give surfactant. If intubating on the neonatal unit (NNU) consider intubation drugs.
B	Breathing	If spontaneously breathing consider CPAP. If apnoeic or poor respiratory effort use a T-piece resuscitator if available and an appropriate size mask. Start with a PIP of 25 and use PEEP of around 5. If chest movement is obvious consider an early reduction in PIP. Start with 30% oxygen, titrate according to saturations. Is remaining on CPAP an option? Is a less invasive surfactant administration (LISA) an option? If intubated give surfactant.
C	Circulation	Support the circulation whilst avoiding excessive volume resuscitation.
D	Disability	Minimise risk factors for intraventricular haemorrhage for example labile blood pressure.
E	Exposure	Maintain good thermal care. Minimise handling.
F	Family	Remember this is likely to be a stressful, distressing time for the family. Explain what is happening to their baby.

Use of CPAP at birth for extremely preterm babies

Newborn preterm babies may be assisted in their transition to air breathing using nasal continuous positive airways pressure (CPAP) rather than routine intubation. Early use of nasal CPAP should be considered in those spontaneously breathing infants who are at risk of developing respiratory distress syndrome (RDS). CPAP can be delivered by face mask or nasal prongs, however CPAP is not always possible for the smallest, least mature babies e.g. < 25 weeks. CPAP has been shown to be better than humidified high-flow oxygen as a primary mode of respiratory support at birth.

Surfactant

Surfactant is an important treatment that improves survival and reduces pneumothoraces. The European consensus guideline on RDS suggests an overall aim should be to avoid invasive mechanical ventilation, if possible, whilst endeavouring to give surfactant as early as possible in the course of RDS once it is deemed necessary.

An animal derived surfactant should be given to any extremely preterm baby who is intubated on labour ward or as part of their early care on the neonatal unit. For extremely preterm babies stabilised on CPAP, surfactant should be given if the oxygen requirement is > 30% whilst using a PEEP of at least 6 cm H_2O.

Most surfactants have similar efficacy when used in similar doses; however, there is a survival advantage when 200 mg kg^{-1} of poractant alfa is given compared with 100 mg kg^{-1} of beractant or 100 mg kg^{-1} poractant alfa to treat RDS.

Surfactant administration techniques

Intubation
Correct tracheal tube placement should be confirmed by end-tidal CO_2 detection, bilateral air entry and equal chest rise. Surfactant is then administered down the tracheal tube using an appropriate catheter. Care should be taken that the catheter is not advanced past the tip of the tracheal tube as this may result in unilateral surfactant administration. Surfactant dispersal is aided by positive pressure ventilation and following this, lung compliance should improve and reduction of ventilation pressures should be considered. If volume controlled ventilation is provided, the delivered pressure for a set tidal volume is likely to reduce. Following surfactant, plans for early extubation should be made where possible.

Insure (IN-Sur-E)
This is a technique that involves tracheal intubation, surfactant administration followed by extubation. It aims to avoid ongoing mechanical ventilation following surfactant administration. Patient selection using clinical criteria and blood gases may help indicate which babies are at greater risk of extubation failure.

LISA (Less invasive surfactant administration)
This involves surfactant administration to a baby receiving CPAP. The vocal cords are visualised using laryngoscopy and a suitable catheter is passed through the cords whilst keeping the CPAP delivery device in place. The laryngoscope can be removed once the catheter is in place and surfactant is slowly instilled into the lungs. This technique avoids ongoing mechanical ventilation. It does however require laryngoscopy and this has created debate about the use of sedation for the procedure. There is a balance between sedation that reduces discomfort and

the rise in intracranial pressure that laryngoscopy causes and a level of sedation that may impair respiratory drive. Low doses of sedatives or analgesics such as fentanyl, propofol or midazolam have been studied but optimal dosing regimens have yet to be defined.

Early care of the extremely preterm infant

An extremely preterm baby admitted to the neonatal unit should undergo an ABCDEF assessment on arrival. Following this, good early care requires timely, appropriate interventions and the concept of the 'golden hour' is sometimes used. This is more about timely completion of interventions rather than an absolute target of 60 min. These timely interventions include ensuring the baby is settled onto the chosen mode of respiratory support, weighing the baby, the continuation of good thermal care with temperature checks, cardiorespiratory monitoring, a blood gas including glucose checks, obtaining vascular access, the provision of maintenance fluids and the administration of antibiotics and vitamin K.

After this initial phase further assessment with a cranial ultrasound and echocardiogram (if part of the local management protocol) should be considered. An approach to initial management of an extremely preterm baby is shown in Figure 3.1.

Mechanical ventilation

Mechanical ventilation is invasive ventilation delivered through a tracheal tube. There are multiple modes of mechanical ventilation often with slightly different names according to the ventilator used. The NICE Specialist neonatal respiratory care for babies born preterm guideline recommends using synchronised volume targeted ventilation as a primary mode of invasive ventilator support with high frequency oscillating ventilation if this is not effective. When using volume ventilation, tidal volumes of 4–8 mL kg^{-1} are commonly used. If volume ventilation is not available when transferring an intubated baby from labour ward to the neonatal unit, the minimum pressure needed to achieve adequate, but not excessive, chest movement should be used.

The duration of mechanical ventilation should be minimised and whilst ventilated, the ventilation strategies should be reviewed regularly and respiratory support weaned where possible because mechanical ventilation is associated with ventilator associated lung injuries and bronchopulmonary dysplasia. Similarly, ventilatory aims should be to avoid lung atelectasis whilst also avoiding over distension. Permissive hypercapnia where a moderate elevation in pCO_2 is accepted as long as the pH is acceptable helps reduce volutrauma and barotrauma to the preterm lung.

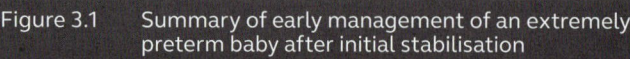

Figure 3.1 Summary of early management of an extremely preterm baby after initial stabilisation

- Transfer to incubator
- Reassess ABCDEF
  Assess level of respiratory support needed
  Apply monitoring
- Surfactant if intubated and not already given
  Avoid excessive chest expansion
- Consider UAC / UVC insertion
  Consider peripheral cannula
  Admission bloods
- IV fluids / TPN
  Medications – IV antibiotics, vitamin K, caffeine
- X-rays for tracheal tube and line positions
- Reassess ABCDEF and blood gases
  Wean ventilation if possible
  Consider early extubation
- Cranial ultrasound
  Echocardiogram if indicated by local policy
  Complete documentation
  Chase blood results
  Update parents

Non-invasive ventilation (NIV)

NIV options include continuous positive airway pressure (CPAP), Bi-level CPAP (BIPAP) or its synchronised alternative (SIPAP) and humidified high-flow nasal cannula oxygen (HHFNC). CPAP is most commonly used as a primary mode of non-invasive ventilation and is recommended in the European consensus guideline on RDS management. Other NIV have been trialled and are generally equivalent to CPAP but have not been shown to be better. CPAP at birth has been shown to be better than HFNC for reducing the need for intubation.

Monitoring

Extremely preterm babies should have continuous monitoring during their early care on the NNU. This would commonly include heart rate, respiratory rate and oxygen saturation. Blood pressure should be recorded either invasively through an arterial line (umbilical or peripheral) or non-invasively.

Intravascular access

Extremely preterm babies require intravascular access and this commonly includes an umbilical venous catheter (UVC) and often an umbilical arterial catheter (UAC). Peripheral venous cannula are regularly used and if UVC access is unavailable a peripherally inserted long line may be needed. These procedures are covered in Chapter 13.

Medications

A number of drugs may need to be prescribed; these include:

First line antibiotics
Local protocols vary but benzylpenicillin and gentamicin are commonly used appropriate first line antibiotics to cover for the possibility of neonatal sepsis (see Chapter 10).

Vitamin K
To reduce the risk of haemorrhagic disease of the newborn.

Caffeine
This is a respiratory stimulant and was shown in the CAP trial to facilitate earlier extubation, reduce bronchopulmonary dysplasia and lead to better neurodevelopmental outcomes at 18 months.
At 11 years old, caffeine-treated children had better respiratory function and reduced risk of motor impairment compared to those who did not receive caffeine.

Management of the ductus arteriosus

It is normal for the ductus arteriosus to be open at birth; its persistent patency can sometimes become problematic over time due to high pulmonary blood flow, pulmonary oedema and volume loading of the heart. Treatments can be conservative, medical or surgical and approaches to treatment can be prophylactic, targeted prophylaxis or expectant. Targeted prophylaxis for ductal management requires relatively early echocardiography and medical treatment often with ibuprofen or paracetamol. Optimal ductal management remains unclear and research is ongoing; local unit protocols should be followed.

Thermoregulation

Maintaining normothermia (temperature 36.5–37.5°C) is important in the preterm infant because low temperatures are associated with increased morbidity and mortality. Attention to thermoregulation is vital from the time of delivery to neonatal unit admission and thereafter. The use of plastic bags at delivery in conjunction with an overhead heater and incubator humidity are all important. Care must be taken when transferring the baby and when performing procedures in the initial stabilisation period to ensure that normothermia is maintained.

Nutrition

Early parenteral nutrition should be used where appropriate and enteral feeds started early, preferably with maternal colostrum; local unit protocols should be followed.

Progress and prognosis

Risks of survival and disability are commonly considered in the context of antenatal counselling. However, with the knowledge of how stable a baby has been on the neonatal unit, this assessment should be updated. There is a concept of developmental trajectories so that two identical babies with the same survival and disability risks at birth may have very different outlooks a week later or at 36 weeks corrected age depending on postnatal events. Figure 3.2 illustrates this concept.

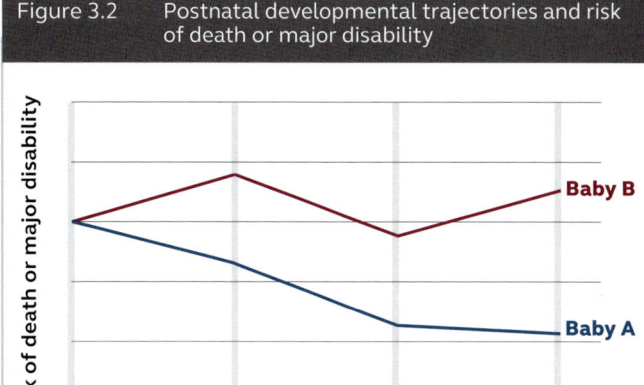

Figure 3.2 Postnatal developmental trajectories and risk of death or major disability

Baby A
A 24 week gestation, 700 g birthweight baby, ventilated for 12 h, one dose surfactant followed by successful extubation to CPAP.

At 7 days old they were weaning CPAP and establishing enteral feeding.

They were off respiratory support and gaining weight well by 28 days.

At 36 weeks corrected age they were breast feeding, growing well, had a normal cranial ultrasound and no retinopathy of prematurity.

Baby B
A 24 week gestation, 700 g birthweight baby, two doses of surfactant, pulmonary haemorrhage on day 2, and a left-sided grade 4 IVH on day 4.

They were ventilated for 2 weeks followed by 6 weeks CPAP.

At 28 days old they had medically managed NEC requiring ventilation for 4 days.

They had bilateral laser treatment for ROP and at 36 weeks were preparing for discharge with supplemental home oxygen.

03: Summary learning

Optimal antenatal care, including delivery at an appropriate centre, improves outcomes.

Antenatal counselling should be informed, relevant, honest and clear.

Management of the extremely preterm infant at birth requires careful planning and often gentle stabilisation and assistance of transition rather than resuscitation.

Timely interventions after admission to NNU help with ongoing stabilisation.

Minimising invasive ventilation and use of non-invasive respiratory support where possible is associated with better outcomes.

Parental updates are vitally important and parents should continue to be updated about their baby's postnatal progress.

In an extremely preterm baby that does not need immediate resuscitation delayed cord clamping improves survival.

My key take-home messages from this chapter are:

Further reading

Ambalavanan N, Carlo WA, Tyson JE, Langer JC, Walsh MC, Parikh NA, Das A, Van Meurs KP, Shankaran S, Stoll BJ, Higgins RD; Generic Database; Subcommittees of the Eunice Kennedy Shriver National Institute of Child Health and Human Development Neonatal Research Network. Outcome trajectories in extremely preterm infants. Pediatrics. 2012 Jul;130(1):e115-25. doi: 10.1542/peds.2011-3693. Epub 2012 Jun 11. PMID: 22689874; PMCID: PMC3382921.

Adams-Chapman I, Heyne R, DeMauro S, et al.; Follow-Up Study of the Eunice Kennedy Shriver National Institute of Child Health and Human Development Neonatal Research Network. Neurodevelopmental impairment among extremely preterm infants in the Neonatal Research Network. Pediatrics. 2018;141:e20173091.

British Association of Perinatal Medicine. Perinatal Management of Extreme Preterm Birth before 27 weeks of gestation A Framework for Practice October 2019 https://hubble-live-assets.s3.amazonaws.com/bapm/attachment/file/182/Extreme_Preterm_28-11-19_FINAL.pdf

Chawla S, Natarajan G, Shankaran S, Carper B, Brion LP, Keszler M, et al.; Eunice Kennedy Shriver National Institute of Child Health and Human Development Neonatal Research Network. Markers of successful extubation in extremely preterm infants, and morbidity after failed extubation. J Pediatr. 2017 Oct;189:113–119.e2.

Ding S, Lemyre B, Daboval T, Barrowman N, Moore G. A meta-analysis of neurodevelopmental outcomes at 4-10 years in children born at 22-25 weeks gestation. Acta Paediatr. 2019;108(7):1237–44.

Doyle LW, Ranganathan S, Cheong JL. Neonatal caffeine treatment and respiratory function at 11 years in children under 1,251 g at birth. Am J Respir Crit Care Med. 2017 Nov;196(10):1318–24.

Doyle LW, Crowther CA, Middleton P, Marret S, Rouse D. Magnesium sulphate for women at risk of preterm birth for neuroprotection of the fetus. Cochrane Database Syst Rev. 2009 Jan;1(1):CD004661.

Fawke J, Tinnion RJ, Monnelly V, Ainsworth SB, Cusack J, Wyllie J. How does the BAPM Framework for Practice on Perinatal Management of Extreme Preterm Birth Before 27 Weeks of Gestation impact delivery of Newborn Life Support? A Resuscitation Council UK response. Arch Dis Child Fetal Neonatal Ed. 2020 Nov;105(6):672-674. doi: 10.1136/archdischild-2020-318927. Epub 2020 Apr 9. PMID: 32273302.

Johnson S, Fawke J, Hennessy E, Rowell V, Thomas S, Wolke D, Marlow N. Neurodevelopmental disability through 11 years of age in children born before 26 weeks of gestation. Pediatrics. 2009;124:e249–57.

Hughes, RG, Brocklehurst, P, Steer, PJ, Heath, P, Stenson, BM on behalf of the Royal College of Obstetricians and Gynaecologists. Prevention of early-onset neonatal group B streptococcal disease. Green-top Guideline No. 36. BJOG 2017; 124:e280– e305.

Katheria AC, Szychowski JM, Essers J, Mendler MR, Dempsey EM, Schmölzer GM, et al. Early Cardiac and Cerebral Hemodynamics with Umbilical Cord Milking Compared with Delayed Cord Clamping in Infants Born Preterm. J Pediatr. 2020 Aug;223:51-56.e1. doi: 10.1016/j.jpeds.2020.04.010. Epub 2020 May 29. PMID: 32482392; PMCID: PMC7387184.

Marlow N, Bennett C, Draper ES, Hennessy EM, Morgan AS, Costeloe KL. Perinatal outcomes for extremely preterm babies in relation to place of birth in England: the EPICure 2 study. Arch Dis Child Fetal Neonatal Ed. 2014 May;99(3):F181–8.

Moore T, Hennessy E, Myles J, Johnson S, Draper E, Costeloe K, Marlow N. Neurological and developmental outcome in extremely preterm children born in England in 1995 and 2006: the EPICure studies. BMJ. 2012;345:e7961.

National Institute for Health and Care Excellence (NICE) guideline. Specialist neonatal respiratory care for babies born preterm. https://www.nice.org.uk/guidance/ng124

Norman M, Piedvache A, Børch K, Huusom LD, Bonamy AE, Howell EA, et al.; Effective Perinatal Intensive Care in Europe (EPICE) Research Group. Association of short antenatal corticosteroid administration-to-birth intervals with survival and morbidity among very preterm infants: results from the EPICE cohort. JAMA Pediatr. 2017 Jul;171(7):678–86.

Pascal A, Govaert P, Oostra A, Naulaers G, Ortibus E, Van den Broeck C. Neurodevelopmental outcome in very preterm and very-low-birthweight infants born over the past decade: a meta-analytic review. Dev Med Child Neurol. 2018;60:342–55.

Pierrat V, Marchand-Martin L, Arnaud C, et al.; EPIPAGE-2 Writing Group. Neurodevelopmental outcome at 2 years for preterm children born at 22 to 34 weeks' gestation in France in 2011: EPIPAGE-2 cohort study. BMJ. 2017;358:j3448.

Roberts CT, Owen LS, Manley BJ, Frøisland DH, Donath SM, Dalziel KM, et al.; HIPSTER Trial Investigators. Nasal high-flow therapy for primary respiratory support in preterm infants. N Engl J Med. 2016 Sep;375(12): 1142–51.

Roberts D, Brown J, Medley N, Dalziel SR. Antenatal corticosteroids for accelerating fetal lung maturation for women at risk of preterm birth. Cochrane Database Syst Rev. 2017 Mar;3:CD004454.

Schmidt B, Roberts RS, Davis P, Doyle LW, Barrington KJ, Ohlsson A, et al.; Caffeine for Apnea of Prematurity Trial Group. Caffeine therapy for apnea of prematurity. N Engl J Med. 2006 May;354(20):2112–21.

Schmidt B, Roberts RS, Davis P, Doyle LW, Barrington KJ, Ohlsson A, et al.; Caffeine for Apnea of Prematurity Trial Group. Longterm effects of caffeine therapy for apnea of prematurity. N Engl J Med. 2007 Nov; 357(19):1893–902.

Serenius F, Ewald U, Farooqi A, et al; Extremely Preterm Infants in Sweden Study Group. Neurodevelopmental outcomes among extremely preterm infants 6.5 years after active perinatal care in Sweden. JAMA Pediatr 170:954–963.

Singh N, Halliday HL, Stevens TP, Suresh G, Soll R, Rojas-Reyes MX. Comparison of animal-derived surfactants for the prevention and treatment of respiratory distress syndrome in preterm infants. Cochrane Database Syst Rev. 2015 Dec;(12):CD010249.

Sweet D, Carniellib V, Greisen G, Hallmand M, Ozeke E, te Pas A et al. European Consensus Guidelines on the Management of Respiratory Distress Syndrome – 2019 Update. Neonatology 2019;115:432–450 DOI: 10.1159/000499361.

WHO. WHO recommendations on interventions to improve preterm birth outcomes. Geneva: WHO; 2015.

Wyckoff MH, Weiner GM, et al. Neonatal Life Support 2020 International Consensus on Cardiopulmonary Resuscitation and Emergency Cardiovascular Care Science With Treatment Recommendations. Pediatrics. 2020; doi: 10.1542/peds.2020-038505C.

Recognition of the deteriorating infant   04

In this chapter

Situational awareness and early intervention

Neonatal Early Warning Scores

Rapid relevant clinical observations

Interpreting your findings

Managing identified problems

Putting it all together and decision making

The learning outcomes will enable you to:

Use the ARNI algorithm to assess any baby rapidly and direct immediate management. Decide if their condition is:

- Potentially life-threatening (i.e. they are physiologically unstable and in need of immediate support)
- Worrying: some immediate management is needed, there is cause for concern
- Satisfactory

Use an ABC approach for immediate management, followed by regular ABCDEF reassessment

Use Neonatal Early Warning Scores

Understand the need for early effective help

Introduction

The newborn infant's condition can change rapidly and can be difficult to assess, even for experienced practitioners. During the transition from fetal to infant life, behaviour or physical signs that would be abnormal at other times may be normal.

For instance, the normal term baby may have blue hands and feet on the first day and sleep deeply for several hours. How do we distinguish this from unconsciousness and circulatory failure? Conversely, the signs of abnormality may be subtle and easily missed; life-threatening sepsis may present as tachypnoea with some expiratory grunting.

Prevention

The goal is to prevent deterioration. The newborn, especially if preterm, has a limited ability to deal with physiological stress. Neonatal care is often directed at maintaining homeostasis. For instance, the incubator is designed to help a baby maintain a correct body temperature and avoid the metabolic cost of either hypo or hyperthermia. Babies who become cold may develop hypoxia, metabolic acidosis and produce less lung surfactant and are significantly more likely to die. Skilled nursing will provide the baby with an environment which minimises stress and responds to early indications of discomfort.

However, not all deterioration is preventable and we need a method of rapidly assessing babies which identifies those who are ill or in need of support, without medicalising normal babies. This chapter presents a structured approach to assessment of the newborn about which there is concern.

The approach is based on:

- situational awareness and early intervention
- relevant clinical observations
- clear documentation of observations
- decisive action.

Situational awareness

The term situational awareness originates from the military and is frequently used in aviation, meaning to understand what is going on around you. For a baby it means the team having an understanding of the whole clinical picture including previous antenatal and perinatal history and likely developments. It requires an ability to sift information rapidly and focus on important risks whilst remaining aware of the whole picture. This is covered in more detail in Chapter 5.

In the context of recognition of the deteriorating infant, situational awareness gives an idea as to which babies are at greater risk of deteriorating and increases the chance of noticing quickly when this is happening.

For example, a term baby who has had resuscitation with inflation and ventilation breaths may appear well at 15 min of age. However, the need for resuscitation at birth suggests they may have used some of their glycogen stores and is at risk of hypoglycaemia. They may also be at risk of having sustained hypoxic-ischaemic damage to major organs.

More detailed consideration of the situation (e.g. labour history, cord blood gases, birth weight) helps to refine this risk assessment. Consider the two contrasting case histories below:

Case 1	Evidence of severe fetal compromise (terminal bradycardia on CTG, cord pH < 7.0) with poor condition at birth (HR < 60 bpm and chest compressions needed).
	Risk assessment: very high.
	Admit the baby to the neonatal unit for intensive care and consider neuroprotective cooling.
Case 2	CTG briefly non-reassuring, the cord pH was > 7.2 and baby responded quickly to inflation and ventilation breaths.
	Risk assessment: low to moderate.
	Plan for the baby to remain with the mother under close observation. Keep this baby warm: hypothermia consumes energy which will use up his already depleted reserves. Encourage skin to skin contact with their mother so that when they are physiologically ready they can go to the breast where colostrum will provide some fuel. It is likely that these simple physiological measures will help keep this baby clinically stable and avoid a downward spiral of hypothermia, hypoglycaemia and respiratory distress.

Clinical decision making tools e.g. newborn early warning scores (NEWS) or standardised sepsis calculators can help improve consistency in situational awareness, aid early intervention and prevention of neonatal infection (see Chapter 10).

Neonatal early warning scores (NEWS)

Be clear about the nature and frequency of observations you request and what to do if they are abnormal. If the baby described in Case 2 did deteriorate, awareness that you might observe hypoglycaemia, seizures or cardiorespiratory problems would increase your alertness to relevant clinical signs.

When babies are having regular clinical observations; whether in intensive care or on a maternity ward, you must record the observations in a way which helps you interpret and act on them. Early warning scores have been developed and validated in acutely ill adult, obstetric and paediatric patients and this principle can be applied to the newborn.

These early warning scores promote two important safety principles: early recognition of a potential problem and sharing any concerns. These scores are best viewed as useful clinical tools rather than precision instruments with known sensitivity and specificity.

An example of a neonatal early warning score suitable for use with relatively well babies on maternity wards is shown in Figure 4.1. it is easy to see if any observations fall in the coloured part of the chart. The chart is accompanied by guidance on a graded response depending on the number of highlighted observations. This helps relatively junior members of staff to be assertive in escalating potential problems.

Interpretation

The first question is whether your observations are normal or abnormal, given the baby's situation. Decision aids, such as the early warning charts described above, are very useful. These decision aids help protect you from 'cognitive errors', meaning the mistakes that humans make during complex information processing. An example is failing to appreciate an abnormal clinical sign because you had already made another diagnosis and were not expecting to see it. The act of plotting a value in the 'coloured' zone increases the chances of you picking up and acting on the abnormal sign.

If the observations are abnormal, you need to quickly identify anything which represents an immediate threat to the baby's life – in other words problems affecting airway, breathing and circulation. Manage problems as you find them and remember that the clinical situation can change quickly and regular reassessment is important.

Figure 4.1 Neonatal Early Warning Score (NEWS) Chart suitable for use for use in maternity wards for babies nursed with their mothers

1. Record observations. 2. Add up shaded boxes (1 point each). 3. Enter Total NEWS 4. Act on Total NEWS

Date											
Time											
Temperature	38										
	37										
	36										
	35										
	34										
Heart rate	200+										
	190										
	180										
	170										
	160										
	150										
	140										
	130										
	120										
	110										
	100										
	90										
	0-89										
	Heart										
SaO$_2$	≥ 95										
	< 95										
Respiratory rate	70+										
	60										
	50										
	40										
	30										
	20										
	0-19										
	Resp Rate										
Respiratory distress	Present										
	Absent										
Prefeed BM	<2.0										
	>2.6										
	BM										
☑ if passed urine											
☑ if passed meconium											
Normal tone & behaviour											
Floppy / jittery / irritable											
Feeding (see chart attached)	Satisfactory										
	Unsatisfactory										
☑ if concerned about patient											
Total NEWS Alert Level	0 / 1-2 / 3+										
Patient Reviewed ☑											

Recognition of the deteriorating infant

Early effective intervention

Early effective intervention involves:

1. Recognising the need for intervention in the first place
2. Rapid clinical assessment
3. Rapid stabilisation
4. Slowing the progression of any illness
5. Avoiding iatrogenic harm.

It is vital to recognise the immediate needs of the baby through an effective structured assessment process. Early effective intervention needs the right people to be in the right place at the right time, with the right equipment, working together.

Initial problems should be identified as quickly as possible, frequent reassessment will facilitate stabilising the baby and diagnosing underlying problems. This early phase of management has often been called 'the Golden Hour'. This concept comes from emergency medicine. The exact timing is less important than ensuring optimal management without delay. Delay can lead to worse outcomes illustrated in Figure 4.2.

Resuscitation

Acute, life-threatening problems need to be dealt with immediately. Applying the standard ABC approach the priorities are (Temperature) Airway, Breathing, Circulation followed by reassessment Thermal care is extremely important, particularly for preterm babies (see Chapter 3).

Stabilisation

Preventing further deterioration, supporting normal physiological parameters and building the foundations for definitive therapy.

Definitive therapy

Instituting the treatment required to treat the underlying problem. The baby moves through resuscitation to stabilisation to definitive therapy via a series of reassessments (Figure 4.3).

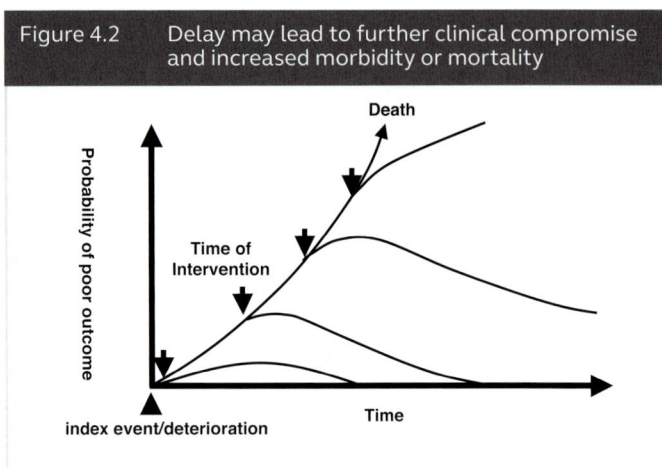

Figure 4.2 Delay may lead to further clinical compromise and increased morbidity or mortality

Initial rapid clinical assessment

When called to assess a baby who is giving cause for concern you should aim to complete a rapid clinical assessment within about one minute. Start with vital signs and the information from monitoring (such as oxygen saturation) which is already in place or is quick to apply.

Useful rapid observations

A Airway

Look at head position, inspect the mouth and nose for the presence of secretions, listen for airway noises.

B Breathing

Respiratory rate, depth and pattern. Synchronisation with ventilator if applicable. Oxygen saturation if monitor already on or immediately available.

C Circulation

Heart rate, central capillary refill time, blood pressure (if equipment already in place).

> Act on any significant problems with ABC before moving on

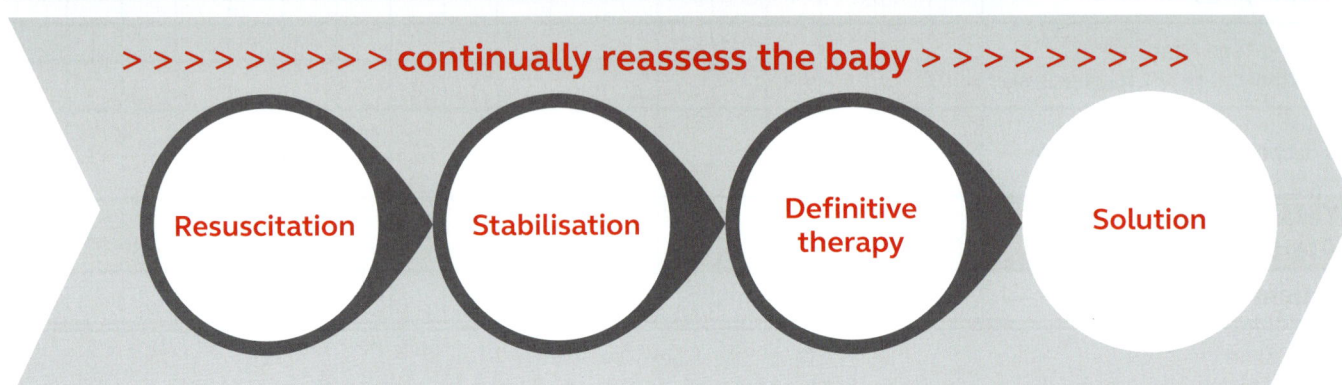

Figure 4.3 Three phases of early effective intervention

Table 4.1 A guide to diagnosing tracheal tube problems in the intubated baby

Observation	Yes / no	Interpretation				
		Tube correct	Tube blocked	Tube displaced	Lungs have become stiffer	Asymmetrical lung disease
Does the chest move with breaths given by the ventilator, T-piece or self inflating bag?	Yes	x				
	No		x	x		
Does chest move only with high pressures?	Yes		x		x	
	No	–	–	–	–	–
Listen in both axillae – is there air entry?	Yes	x				
	No or doubtful		x	x		
Is the air entry exactly the same on both sides?	Yes	x				
	No			x		x
Listen over the stomach – is there a lot of noise with ventilation?	Yes			x		
	No	–	–	–	–	–
NB Clinical assessment of tracheal tube placement and patency can be unreliable. Assessment should be combined with end-tidal capnography to increase accuracy. Remember the DOPE algorithm (see Chapter 7) to troubleshoot tracheal tube problems						

Once ABC are satisfactory or are being dealt with, look for further information. You may have more sophisticated cot-side information such as measures of pressure, volume and flow from a ventilator, end-tidal carbon dioxide ($ETCO_2$), transillumination of the chest via cold light, physiological monitoring (heart rate, saturations, respiratory rate).

Once your rapid ABC assessment and any immediate actions have been completed, you should reassess ABCDEF.

D Disability

Feel the baby's tone and establish responsiveness to normal handling. Check pupillary responses.

D Dextrose

Bedside testing from a capillary sample using a meter designed to detect low values.

E Exposure and everything else

Central temperature – address hypo or hyperthermia, visual inspection of the whole body, capillary blood gases.

F Family

Once you have completed your assessment and initial actions, communicate clearly with the family about what you think at this stage and what you are planning to do. Record conversations you have with the family in the medical record.

The outcome of a clinical review should be documented in the notes with actions clearly recorded e.g.

- Further escalation of review
- Increase in frequency of observations
- Changes in patient management
- Admit to neonatal unit.

> Remember: If you feel you need more help at any time, call for help – regardless of NEWS Score

Interpreting observations and managing problems

A Airway

Baby with no tracheal tube

What is the head position? Babies with airway obstruction may adopt an extended head position. Babies with poor tone may not be able to maintain a neutral position. Support the head in the neutral position if necessary.

Is there any visible obstruction in the mouth? Remove anything you can see with a wide bore suction catheter.

Are there transmitted large airway noises with breathing? If so, try positioning and suction of nose and mouth.

Baby with a tracheal tube

A displaced or obstructed tube could well be the source of the problem. Initial clinical observation can rapidly detect tube problems. If the chest moves with the ventilation system and there is good air entry, the tube is probably satisfactory. Poor chest movement suggests a blocked or displaced tube or a decrease in lung compliance. Asymmetrical air entry suggests a displaced tube or asymmetrical lung disease such as diaphragmatic hernia, collapse of one lung or pneumothorax.

You may have $ETCO_2$ colour change capnography or other physiological measures from the ventilator to assist you. If you can interpret these measures, use them. If you are not familiar with the ventilator outputs, disconnect the ventilator and hand ventilate the baby via a T-piece or self-inflating bag, while someone else checks the ventilator. This immediately bypasses any faults within the ventilator.

The mnemonic **DOPE** (displaced, obstructed, pneumothorax, equipment) can be useful for assessing clinical deterioration in a ventilated baby.

See Table 4.1 for a guide to diagnosing tracheal tube problems.

If you suspect a tube problem you must call for help and act immediately to unblock or replace the tube. If in doubt, take it out and initiate mask ventilation.

B Breathing

Assess the rate, depth and pattern of breathing to assess if breathing is adequate. If the baby is breathing at a normal rate for gestation, the pattern is fairly regular and the chest movement is easily visible, breathing is likely to be satisfactory.

The normal term newborn has a respiratory rate between 40 and 60 breaths per min. Babies who are unconscious or exhausted will breathe too slowly. Babies with abnormal lungs, sepsis, shock, acidosis or cerebral irritability may breathe too fast.

Periodic breathing with short periods of apnoea (up to 5 s) is normal in babies, particularly during sleep in preterms. Longer periods of apnoea with changes in colour, oxygen saturation or heart rate may be a sign of illness and may need intervention.

Look for signs of respiratory distress, including:
- subcostal, sternal and intercostal recession
- nasal flaring
- head bobbing
- tracheal tugging
- expiratory grunting.

Oxygen saturation is best measured from the right arm (reflecting pre-ductal values) and needs to be interpreted in the light of the baby's gestation, postnatal age and previous oxygen requirement. 75% of term babies should have oxygen saturation in the right hand above 90% by 10 min of age. Term babies requiring intervention or ongoing assessment with oxygen saturations below the 25th centile shown in Table 4.2 may require supplemental oxygen.

Table 4.2 Right arm oxygen saturations in term newborn babies

Time from birth	Acceptable (25th centile) right arm saturation
2 min	65%
5 min	85%
10 min	90%

Preterm babies are often monitored and a reduction in oxygen saturation or an increase in the concentration of oxygen needed to maintain saturations are signs of deteriorating lung disease. If you don't have access to a saturation monitor look for central cyanosis, but this is a late clinical sign of hypoxia.

You may have transcutaneous oxygen or CO_2 monitors. Low oxygen and high CO_2 are signs of respiratory failure.

If breathing is very slow, shallow or irregular and/or oxygen saturation cannot be easily maintained above 90%, ventilate the baby via mask and T-piece or self-inflating bag before you go any further.

Transillumination of the chest using a cold light can be done in seconds and is a useful indicator of tension pneumothorax in preterm babies deteriorating to the point of cardiorespiratory failure. This test is more reliable in a darkened environment.

C Circulation

Heart rate

A low heart rate (below 100 bpm) should make you suspect hypoxia. Go back and check that you are happy with airway and breathing. Fast heart rates (above 180 bpm) may be due to fever, medications (especially caffeine or inotropes), pain, developing shock or cardiac arrhythmia.

Blood pressure

After 4 h of age one commonly used acceptable level of mean blood pressure (mmHg) is at or above the gestational age in weeks. If the mean arterial pressure in mmHg is less than the gestation in weeks, then the baby may be hypotensive and in need of volume, inotropic support or sometimes both.

Capillary refill time is less useful in the newborn than in older children. Term babies are usually peripherally shut down in the first few hours of life but should have capillary refill time < 2 s over the sternum. Prolonged central capillary refill in the presence of other signs (e.g. tachycardia) should make you consider circulatory failure. Poor peripheral pulses are another sign of shock and absent or poorly palpable femoral pulses may alert you to cardiac problems.

D Disability

In the newborn, tone is a proxy for conscious level. Normal tone does vary with gestation, with the term newborn having pronounced flexor tone. The baby who is floppy and poorly responsive for their gestational age should be viewed as having a reduced conscious level equivalent to being responsive only to pain. At this level of consciousness, the airway is at risk. Reduced consciousness can be a result of cardiorespiratory failure or reflect a brain problem such as intraventricular haemorrhage.

D Dextrose

Babies are very likely to become hypoglycaemic when unwell. Check blood glucose and give IV dextrose (2.5 mL kg^{-1} 10% dextrose bolus, followed by a dextrose infusion) to any baby who is unwell and whose glucose is ≤ 2.0 mmol. Ensure adequate ongoing glucose delivery, through either feeds or IV fluids, in babies who have needed a glucose bolus for hypoglycaemia.

E Exposure and everything else

Carry out a rapid visual assessment looking at the wider picture for additional clues – think about jaundice, oedema or dehydration, skin rashes, abdominal distension, abnormal nasogastric aspirates, abnormal stools, lumps or red areas on trunk or limbs, swellings on the head or abnormal fontanelle. What indwelling tubes or lines does the baby have? Chest drains can slip or block, long lines can cause cardiac tamponade. These clues may assist you with a definitive diagnosis after the initial period of stabilisation.

Unless you have decided to implement therapeutic hypothermia, take active steps to maintain the temperature of the newly born infant between 36.5°C and 37.5°C. Non-therapeutic hypothermia increases mortality.

You may be able to check blood gases. This will detect hypoxia, hypercapnia, respiratory or metabolic acidosis. Many machines also give other outputs such as lactate, electrolytes, and haematocrit. Make sure you have looked at and used all the information available – remember to maintain your situational awareness.

F Family

Remember that parents will be very anxious when their baby is unwell. Once you have carried out your initial stabilisation, update the family using simple clear language (see Chapter 6).

The ABCDEF approach to initial assessment is summarised in Table 4.3.

Table 4.3 Rapid ABCDEF assessment of baby causing concern

		Rapid ABC	ABCDEF reassessment
A	Airway non intubated	Neutral head position Visible secretions Airway noises	
	Airway intubated	Chest movement and air entry when being ventilated ETCO$_2$	Ventilator outputs ETCO$_2$
B	Breathing	Respiratory rate Chest movement Air entry Apnoea Oxygen saturation	Cold light transillumination
C	Circulation	Heart rate Capillary refill time Blood pressure	Blood pressure
D	Disability Dextrose		Blood glucose Tone and responsiveness
E	Exposure and everything else		Central temperature Inspection of whole body Blood gases
F	Family		Update the family about your plans

ETCO$_2$, oxygen saturation and blood pressure may not be available at first.

Putting it all together – interpretation with initial action

Your aim is to decide if the baby is well or unwell; this will include whether their condition is:

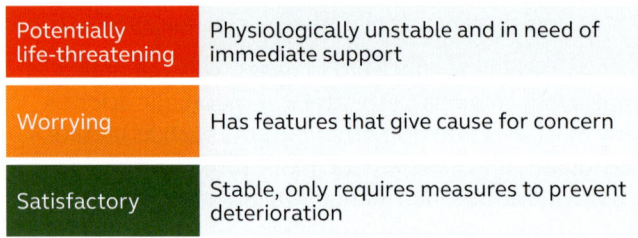

This approach is shown in the ARNI algorithm (Figure 4.5).

Life-threatening features

Babies approaching cardiopulmonary failure will have one or more of the following features:

- obstructed airway
- low oxygen saturation or cyanosis even in supplementary oxygen
- severe respiratory distress
- apnoea or very irregular breathing
- heart rate below 100 bpm
- poor peripheral perfusion
- markedly reduced tone and responsiveness.

For these babies call for help and start life support immediately.

Further ABCDEF assessment

Once life support measures have been started, an ABCDEF assessment can provide further understanding of the cause of cardiopulmonary failure and can direct further life support measures.

The most common neonatal cardiorespiratory arrest rhythm is asystole. The most common precursor is hypoxia due to respiratory failure. As in cardiac arrest in children and adults remember the 4 Hs and 4 Ts (Figure 4.4).

The ABCDEF approach outlined above will pick up pointers to these reversible causes.

Figure 4.4 Reversible causes of cardiac arrest (4 Hs and 4 Ts)

The 4 Hs	The 4 Ts
Hypoxia	Tension pneumothorax
Hypovolaemia	Tamponade (cardiac)
Hypo / hyperkalaemia / metabolic	Toxins
Hypothermia	Thrombosis (coronary or pulmonary)

The ARNI approach to rapid assessment and immediate management of the baby about who is deteriorating or about which there is concern is summarised in Figure 4.3.

Calling for help

When babies deteriorate, they need skilled help quickly. Always ask for help early. Inexperienced clinicians need senior help. Experienced team leaders need a number of helpers so that various actions can be carried out simultaneously and they can stand back and lead.

How to call for help

In the peri-arrest situation put out an emergency call using whatever the local arrangements are. Know the cardiac arrest number (2222 in UK & European hospitals) and know how the team you want is described in your institution. There may be separate paediatric and neonatal teams in large centres. If you are asking someone else to put out the call be very clear with your instructions. Tell them the number to dial, the team to call and the precise location.

If the situation is less serious you may still need help and advice. There are various handover/escalation tools which help with concise and assertive communication.

SBAR (Situation, Background, Assessment, Recommendation) is one such tool and is described in Chapter 5.

Never be afraid to ask for help. The clearer you are about the help you need, the easier it is for someone to assist you.

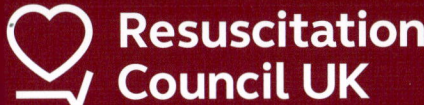

Advanced resuscitation of the newborn infant

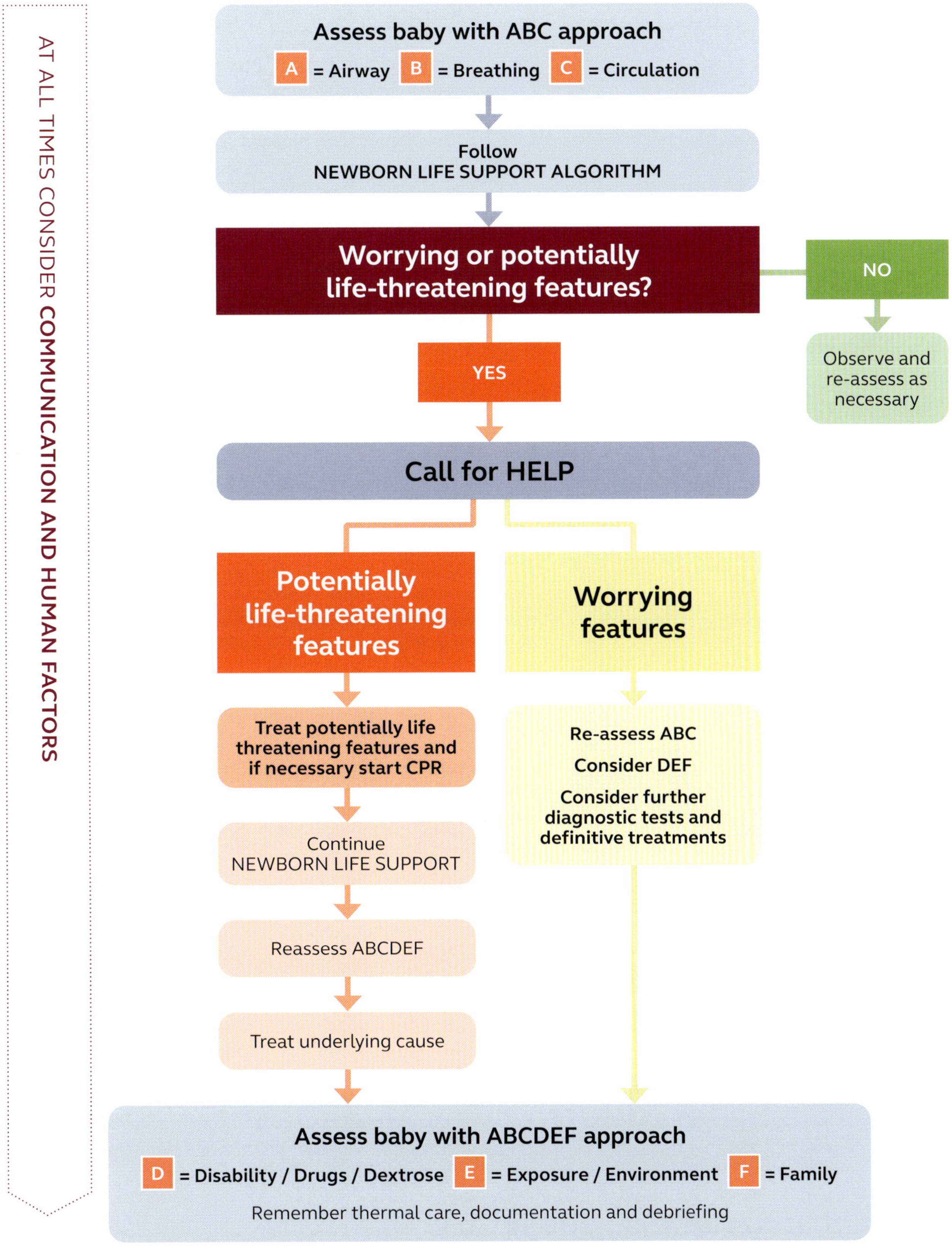

AT ALL TIMES CONSIDER COMMUNICATION AND HUMAN FACTORS

Assess baby with ABC approach
A = Airway   B = Breathing   C = Circulation

↓

Follow NEWBORN LIFE SUPPORT ALGORITHM

↓

Worrying or potentially life-threatening features?

— NO → Observe and re-assess as necessary

— YES ↓

Call for HELP

↓

Potentially life-threatening features | **Worrying features**

Potentially life-threatening features:
- Treat potentially life threatening features and if necessary start CPR
- Continue NEWBORN LIFE SUPPORT
- Reassess ABCDEF
- Treat underlying cause

Worrying features:
- Re-assess ABC
- Consider DEF
- Consider further diagnostic tests and definitive treatments

↓

Assess baby with ABCDEF approach
D = Disability / Drugs / Dextrose   E = Exposure / Environment   F = Family

Remember thermal care, documentation and debriefing

Figure 4.5   ARNI algorithm for assessment and management of baby causing concern

My key take-home messages from this chapter are:

04: Summary learning

Use a rapid ABC approach with immediate interventions followed by an assessment of ABCDEF.

Interpret your findings to categorise if the baby has worrying or life threatening features.

It is important to start interventions to stabilise ABC as soon as you detect problems.

Life support then proceeds in parallel with further re-assessment of ABC, followed by DEF for a definitive diagnosis.

Reassess regularly with an ABCDEF approach.

Call for appropriate help early and use effective concise methods of communication in emergencies.

Further reading

Annibale DJ, David J, Bissinger RL et al. The Golden Hour. Advances in Neonatal care 2010 Vol 10 No 5 p221-223.

Newborn Early Warning Trigger & Track (NEWTT) - a Framework for Practice (2015). A BAPM Framework for Practice https://www.bapm.org/resources/38-newborn-early-warning-trigger-track-newtt-a-framework-for-practice-2015

Dawson JA, Kamlin COF, Vento M et al. Defining the reference range for oxygen saturation in infants after birth. Pediatrics 2010; 125: e1340-7.

Macintosh M, ed. CESDI. Project 27/28. An enquiry into quality of care and its effect on the survival of babies born at 27-28 weeks. London: The Stationery Office, 2003.

McGauhey J, Alderice F, Fowler R, Kapila R, Mayhew A, Moutray M. Outreach and Early Warning Systems (EWS) for the prevention of Intensive Care admission and death of critically ill adult patients on general hospital wards. Cochrane Database Syst Rev. 2007; (3): CD005529.

Norman GR, Eva KW. Diagnostic error and clinical reasoning. Med Educ. 2010; 44(1): 94-100.

Parshuram CS, Duncan HP, Joffe AR et al. Multicentre validation of the bedside paediatric early warning system score: a severity of illness score to detect evolving critical illness in hospitalised children. Crit Care 2011; 15(4): R184.

Pejovic B, Peco-Antic A, Marinkovic-Eric J. Blood pressure in non-critically ill preterm and full-term neonates. Pediatr Nephrol 2007; 22: 249-257.

Tin W. Systolic blood pressure in babies of less than 32 weeks gestation in the first year of life. Northern Neonatal Nursing Initiative. Arch Dis Child Fetal Neonatal Ed 1999; 80: F38-F42.

Communication, human factors and team working

In this chapter

Communication – description of a structured communication tool: Situation, Background, Assessment, Recommendation (SBAR)

Introduction to human factors

The learning outcomes will enable you to:

Understand how to use a structured communication tool to improve sharing information

Gain insight into human factors which may be important in delivering effective care

Introduction

This chapter aims to explore those factors which can impact upon the effective management of critical events. The importance of communication and human factors mean they are central to the ARNI algorithm.

Communication

When dealing with any critical event it is important that team members are able to communicate effectively between themselves and with others. The language of neonatal care and resuscitation is complex. The use of a common language enhances communication and understanding.

In addition to understanding the words used and their context, having a set of tools to frame any communication helps teams to focus on the most important and relevant pieces of information. One of the purposes of the ARNI course is to provide a common framework for structured communication. Situation, Background, Assessment, and Recommendation (SBAR) as described below is one example of a structured communication tool that is widely used in the UK.

SBAR – a structured communication tool

SBAR is a communication tool that has been developed to provide a structure to exchange information in a critical situation. It has a number of potential advantages as it:
- provides a common platform across all disciplines
- ensures clarity when dealing with clinical situations
- streamlines communication and saves time.

SBAR is split into four domains as shown in Table 5.1.

Table 5.1 SBAR – structured communication tool

SBAR	
Situation	The HEADLINE Who are you? Where are you (If not face-to-face)? Who are you talking about? Why are you calling?
Background	Information relevant to the current problem such as: – reason for admission – current diagnoses/problems – drugs – investigations – procedures/therapy.
Assessment	Relevant structured clinical findings, observations, early warning scores. How these are changing, potential interpretation.
Recommendation	What is needed next – such as: – physical help – advice – specific therapeutic interventions.

Table 5.2 Example of 'SBAR'

SBAR example	
Situation	*Hello, this is Sister Jones I am calling from the NICU. I am concerned about baby Smith who has deteriorated on CPAP. Their saturations are 80% on 70% oxygen.*
Background	*They are a 3 day old, 28 week gestation baby who has been on nasal CPAP PEEP 7 cm H20 from birth. They are on antibiotics and TPN via a long line and started feeds yesterday. This morning they received a blood transfusion because their haemoglobin was 95 g L^{-1}.*
Assessment	*They are looking pale and have a markedly increased work of breathing. Their respiratory rate is 80, heart rate is 170, and saturations are 80%. Their mean non-invasive blood pressure is 25 mmHg. I've suctioned milk from their pharynx just now and I wonder if they have aspirated. I've increased the inspired oxygen to 70% and stopped the feed. I'm waiting for a blood gas and sugar.*
Recommendation	*I would like you to come and assess urgently, please. I am concerned they may need ventilation.*

The SBAR tool ensures that whoever is being spoken to has a clear idea of the problem, what the findings are, what is being done, and what is needed next.

In the SBAR example (Table 5.2) note the lack of superfluous information, the relevant information is presented succinctly, and the recommendation is brief and specific.

Some people like to describe 'SBAR and SBAR' – the second SBAR standing for 'stand back and repeat'

Human factors

A widely used definition of human factors is

"Enhancing clinical performance through an understanding of the effects of teamwork, tasks, equipment, workspace, culture and organisation on human behaviour and abilities and application of that knowledge in clinical settings."

Adapted from the Clinical Human Factors Group

Practically, these elements can be described in 4 main categories (Figure 5.1):
1. Systems
2. Processes
3. Procedures
4. Team working, human behaviour and abilities.

1. Systems

Understanding the systems within which we deliver care improves how we are able to do this.

Knowledge of your local physical environment and equipment is essential. How your local service integrates within the neonatal network and transport services is key as well as the location and availability of specialist services a baby may require.

The structure of services and culture in any care setting is part of the care system and effective care is best delivered in an environment that is organised with clear lines of accountability and organisational values that promote learning and improvement.

Knowledge of the systems in which you are delivering care will help with effective care planning – particularly in an emergency situation. Good planning prevents problems. If the systems in place are inadequate, failure to deliver effective care is more likely as the margins for error are reduced. For example, if your labour ward is located on a different floor to the NICU and there is a reliance on a lift to get to babies from labour ward to NICU this will increase clinical risk to the baby in transit from delay, equipment failure or isolation and makes a small issue with a baby more likely to become a significant issue.

2. Processes

When managing an emergency, a process needs to be followed. For instance, adhering to an agreed algorithm (e.g. NLS) or guideline. If everyone knows the expected process, then they are aligned and working together. They are more likely to recognise what is required, anticipate needs and recognise omissions in clinical management. Knowledge of the processes helps ensure the management is appropriate, systematic and timely. Many services use prompts for clinical emergency situations e.g. resuscitation guidelines, checklists or specialised mobile phone applications with doses, lengths of tracheal tubes, infusion calculators etc. These help streamline emergency processes and reduce the risk of errors from cognitive burden in an emergency.

3. Procedures

Management of many clinical situations require interventions or procedures, such as mask inflation, intubation, suction, intravenous cannula insertion, placement of a chest drain. These practical procedures require the right person to be in the right place at the right time with the right equipment and the right support team. An example of this might be intubation – you need someone who has the skill in the right place with the appropriate laryngoscope, tracheal tube, suction etc. and team to assist.

4. Team working, human behaviours and abilities

There are a number of non-technical skills that enable effective team working. Until relatively recently little attention has been paid to these factors in medicine. It is increasingly clear that the way we think, make decisions, communicate and behave in clinical teams is of critical importance to effective care.

There are many systems for examining elements of team working, human behaviours and abilities, here we are going to describe:

- situational awareness
- leadership and active followership
- decision making and cognition
- communication skills
- task management
- errors and being wrong.

Situational awareness

This describes an awareness of what is going on around you. It requires an ability to sift information rapidly and focus on what is important whilst maintaining a global overview, often called the 'helicopter view', of a situation. Ideally an individual clinician has a complete helicopter

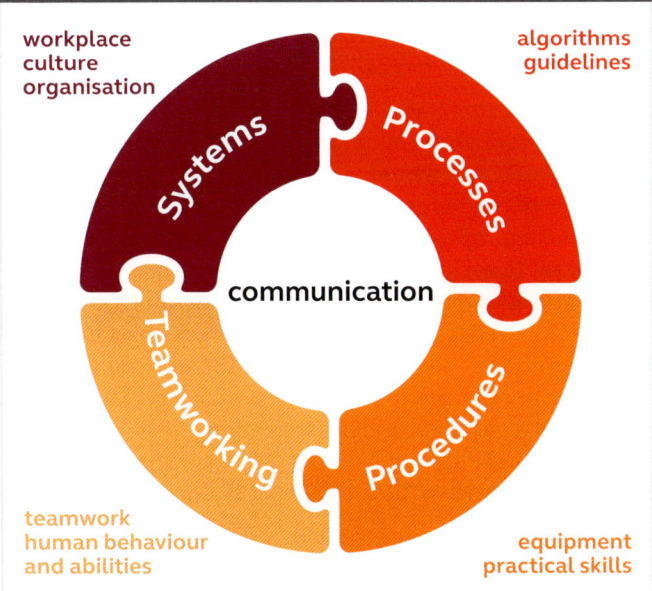

Figure 5.1   An illustration of human factors

view of the overall picture in any given situation and can share this clearly with the team. However, every individual has a limit to what they can hold in their working memory and every individual's working memory capacity is reduced by stress, fatigue, and interruptions. This working memory can be likened to a computer's bandwidth. This analogy is helpful because computers fail to process when their bandwidth is full and this happens to our thinking when we are overloaded with information or stressed. It is easy to see how it is very challenging to maintain situational awareness in a complex situation.

Team working is important in maintaining situational awareness. Each team member has 'bandwidth' to share. An example of this might be a team member noticing deteriorating clinical sign e.g. low saturations that the team leader is unaware of as they are absorbed with deciding a path of action or allocating team roles in a crisis.

In neonatal emergencies we often have very small teams in attendance – sometimes just 2 doctors and a nurse and it is not unusual for a doctor in this situation to have to undertake a manual task, such as intubation. This will reduce their bandwidth and increases the risk of loss of situational awareness. This is why it is best practice to have a team leader who has no manual tasks to complete, whose job is to stand back and take the helicopter view of an event whenever possible. When this is not possible it is important for the other team members to try to maintain situational awareness.

The opposite of situational awareness is fixation. This term is used to describe a situation where specific events achieve a disproportionate and inappropriate significance, diverting the team's attention and resources. An example of this would be concentrating on repeated attempts at intubation at the expense of falling saturations and bradycardia when pausing to provide bag valve mask ventilation to maintain oxygenation would be safer.

The ability to step back and review in a systematic manner is a critical role of the all team members – particularly the team leader. A 'systems check' is a verbal check with members of the team to clarify the current situation and make appropriate plans. This encourages feedback from other team members who often have pertinent observations to make. This is especially helpful if the systems check uses a recognised system, such as the ARNI algorithm, talking through the ABCDEF out loud will often elicit help from those present, will help maintain situational awareness and avoid fixation.

Leadership and active followership

Teams need to be organised with a clear leader. The role of team leader is dynamic and depends on the skill mix and number in the team. Team leadership should not be automatically conferred to the most senior or the most experienced team member but should be given to the person with the skills that enable them to best lead that team in that situation. Who is team leader must be explicitly stated, not implied, and leadership can change during a situation if required.

Active followership is a very important concept in team working. Followership describes team members who are actively maintaining their own situational awareness and actively contributing to the event and sharing their bandwidth. An example of this is when a team member may have a specific piece of information e.g. a blood gas result that the wider team are not aware of. Good followership would be to attract the team leader's attention; perhaps using their name or eye contact (waiting for an appropriate moment) asking if the team leader is ready to receive new information and then clearly stating the result of the gas. Another example of good followership would be if a situation was difficult or the diagnosis was not clear to suggest a recap and reassessment along ABCDEF lines to support the team in all thinking together to help solve the problem.

Attributes of an effective team leader

The team leader should be aware of their limitations and leadership style. They need to:
- maintain a helicopter view
- prioritise tasks
- allocate resources and delegate roles clearly
- call for help if needed
- moderate and control dialogue
- listen to those around whose input and observations may be invaluable
- reassess regularly and rectify problems
- deal with any conflict
- maintain a strategic overview of everything and plan ahead.

Decision-making and cognitive bias

It is important that clear decisions are made, communicated and carried out in a timely manner.

It is important to understand some specific influences on our decision making; these influences are known as cognitive biases.

Cognitive biases are systematic errors in thinking that affect decisions and judgements and are based on a natural tendency to perceive information based on experience and preferences. We are all prone to bias and cannot avoid it completely. However, improving our awareness of types of bias will help us minimise the impact of these natural biases. A full description of bias is outside the scope of the manual but some common examples of bias are described below.

Anchoring bias is when we focus on one particular symptom, sign or piece of information and therefore do not consider others. For example, a jittery baby born to a substance misusing mother being considered to have neonatal abstinence syndrome and not being investigated for hypoglycaemia.

Confirmation bias is looking to confirm a finding that you are expecting. An example of when this is likely is when someone asks you to review a finding that they think is normal and describe to you as being normal. The suggestion of a finding being normal can influence your interpretation of that finding and makes you more likely to agree that the finding is normal.

Availability bias is when we favour the most readily recalled diagnosis. It is especially common if we have encountered this condition recently and if the case affected you greatly. An example of this might be that you have recently seen a severe case of necrotising enterocolitis (NEC) where the baby rapidly deteriorated and died. This experience could influence your decision making and make you more likely to make a diagnosis of NEC and start treatment for this condition in more babies you see subsequently with abdominal distension.

There are many other types of bias that affect our decision making. We are unable to avoid bias in our thinking completely, however, the more aware you are of bias the more able you are to recognise it and reconsider actions you take in light of this understanding. Sharing your mental model and trying to avoid looking only for information that confirms your bias is helpful, as is understanding the impact recent cases have had on you.

Communication within the team

We have already considered how adopting a structured tool such as SBAR can aid handover between individuals and teams. Clear communication between team members is vital during the management of a critical event and team working and effective care is hindered without good communication.

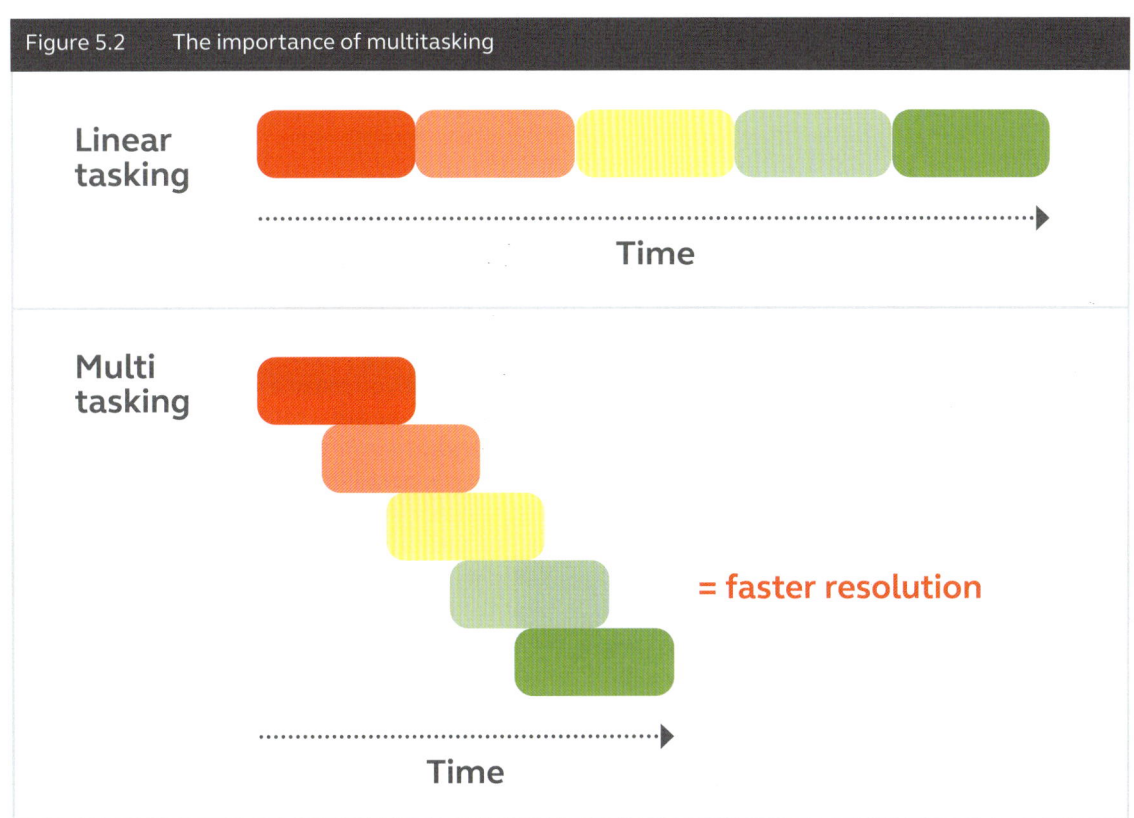

Figure 5.2　The importance of multitasking

Communication in an emergency event should be via the team leader where possible as they need to be aware of what is going on at all times to maintain the helicopter view.

Voices should not be raised. Dialogue should be civil, instructions and questions should be directed to specific people, ideally by name and with precision. Team members should be encouraged to speak if they feel they have something relevant to say – the strength of the team approach is to acknowledge input from all sources. Even the most junior member of staff may have something important to say, and should not be discouraged from saying it.

It is very important to avoid abbreviations or acronyms in emergency events and to use plain language wherever possible. For example, a TOF could be a Tetralogy of Fallot or a Trache-oesophageal Fistula!

Closed loop communication

Closed loop communication is a term that describes when the receiver of information repeats key elements back to the giver of the information. This process ensures that key messages are received and understood and is especially useful in emergency situations.

It is notable that in emergency situations it is common to hear 'can someone get me some adrenaline' or words to that effect. This is not optimal as it is not clear whose responsibility it is to get the adrenaline or how much adrenaline they should prepare. Using a closed loop style of communication as described above will improve the likelihood of the correct dose being made ready as quickly as possible.

For example:

Raj says "Nina can you get me 0.7 mL of 1 in 10 000 adrenaline as quickly as possible please?"

Nina replies "OK, Raj, to confirm you need 0.7 mL of 1 in 10 000 adrenaline urgently. I will get that now and it will be ready in less than 1 minute."

Task management / role allocation

If the team is used effectively then it is possible to optimise management by dealing with more than one issue/problem at a time, accelerating the process and reaching a point of stability and definitive treatment earlier (Figure 5.2).

When there are multiple tasks to undertake it is important to ensure that each task is completed correctly and in a timely manner. Allocating roles and responsibilities for tasks within the team will help share out the tasks and reduce overburdening individuals. It is also very important to prioritise tasks. An example of this might be if a baby needs intubation, IV access and antibiotics. It is most efficient if these tasks are prioritised verbally and allocated to particular team members appropriately. It is important to allocate a team member to help with parent communication and support whenever possible.

Care needs to be taken not to over commit resources, as too large a team may lead to confusion and slower resolution of critical issues. It may also result in reduced cover for other babies already in the neonatal unit as team resources are diverted in other directions. It is the role of the team leader to be aware of this and manage accordingly.

Errors and being wrong

It is the responsibility of everyone involved in dealing with a critical situation to identify any potential errors and communicate via the team leader to enable these to be dealt with effectively. Errors arise as a result of many factors such as ignorance, assumption, misinterpretation, fixation or arrogance:

Ignorance	Not everyone involved may know exactly how to deal with the situation.
Assumption	Ensure that tasks have been completed rather than assuming that they have.
Misinterpretation	Drawing incorrect conclusions from the information available.
Fixation	Focusing exclusively on one aspect of care to the exclusion of other important areas.
Arrogance	Greater self-belief than ability.

If multiple systems fail then problems are compounded and while one failure might have been dealt with, the combination may lead to a crisis.

For example:
Absence of an early warning score may delay recognition of an evolving clinical problem (system).

Methods of summoning an emergency medical team may not work effectively leading to delay in response (system).

An inexperienced emergency team or equipment problems may hinder airway management (procedures/team working).

In this situation multiple events could 'line up' to create a catastrophe which might otherwise have been avoidable. This has been referred to as the 'Swiss cheese' model (Figure 5.3).

Errors are not deliberate; it is very important to appreciate that being wrong 'feels' exactly like being right in the moment that you make a decision. It is only when we find out that we are wrong that we 'feel' wrong and this is always easier with hindsight. We all think we are open to the possibility of being wrong but, in reality, we all genuinely struggle with the reality of admitting we are mistaken. We really need to be actively open to the possibility that we may be wrong by looking for alternative hypotheses, diagnoses, and solutions and by listening carefully and actively entertaining opposing views.

Rehearsal

Rehearsal of situations in advance is a key factor in making systems, teams and individuals as efficient and effective as possible (Figure 5.4).

Practicing in advance allows teams to identify potential problems before they happen, increasing the chances of a successful outcome.

ARNI enables us to rehearse and to learn from mistakes and good practice equally to improve the chance of optimal care in real life crisis situations.

Dealing with a critical event effectively depends on the ability to identify the problem, communicate all relevant details and use resources appropriately.

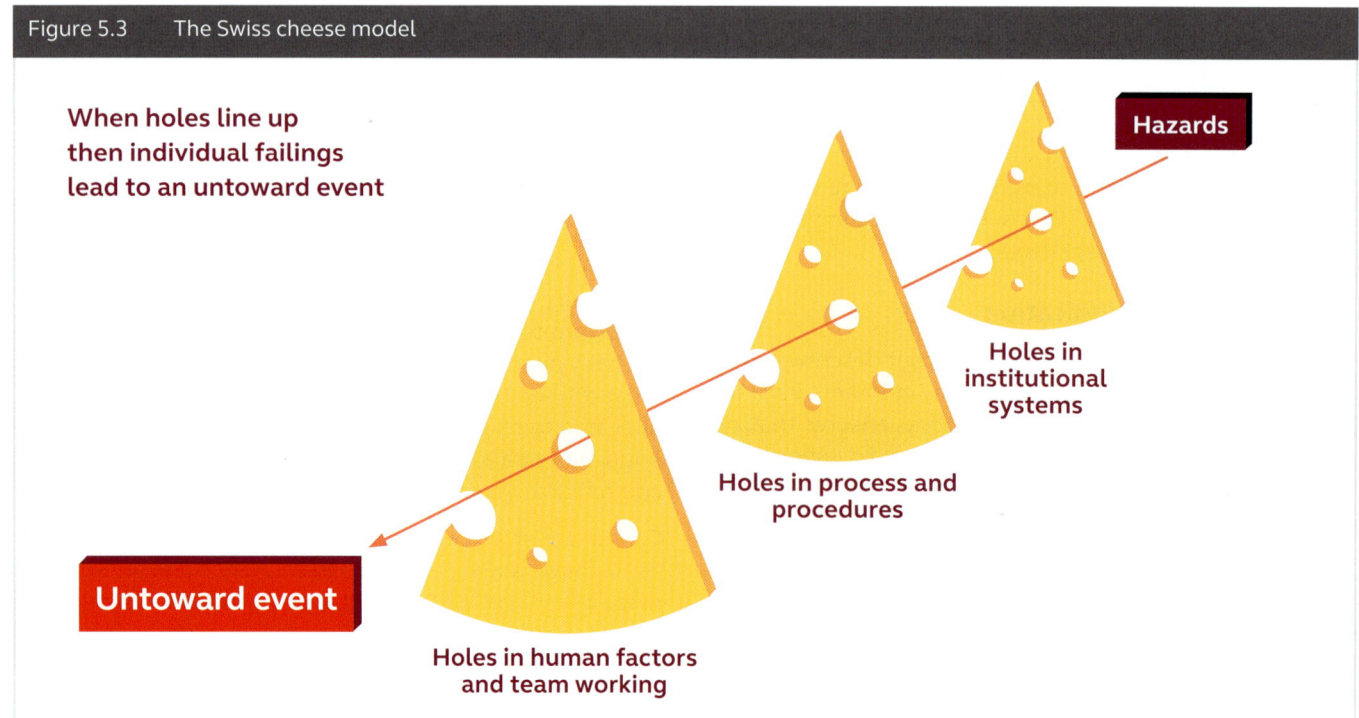

Figure 5.3 The Swiss cheese model

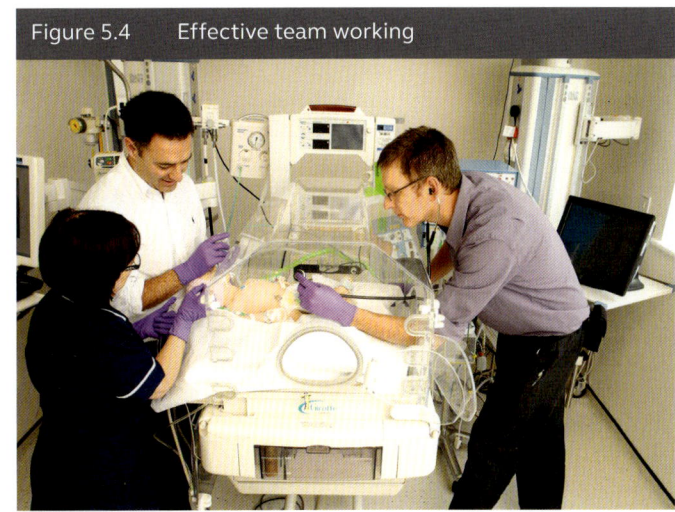

Figure 5.4 Effective team working

SBAR is a useful tool to aid clarity of handover between professionals during critical events.

Managing a critical event effectively requires robust systems, clear processes, competency with practical procedures, unambiguous communication, and leadership and followership and an awareness of the human behaviors and cognitive processes which may influence our ability to manage an event optimally.

Whilst a good outcome can never be guaranteed, having all these elements in place makes success more likely.

05: Summary learning

Dealing with a critical event effectively depends on the ability to identify the problem, communicate all relevant details and use resources appropriately.

SBAR is a useful tool to aid clarity of handover between professionals during critical events.

Managing a critical event effectively requires robust systems, clear processes, competency with practical procedures and unambiguous communication. It also requires leadership, active followership and an awareness of the human behaviors and cognitive processes which may influence our ability to manage an event optimally.

Communication, human factors and team working impact on the effective management of a critical event. Whilst a good outcome can never be guaranteed, having all these elements in place makes success more likely.

My key take-home messages from this chapter are:

Further reading

Advanced Life Support 8th edition. 2021 Resuscitation Council UK. London.

Fioratou E, Flin R, Glavin R. No simple fix for fixation errors: cognitive processes and their clinical applications. Anaesthesia 2010; 65:61-9.

McCrory MC, Aboumatar H, Custer JW, et al. "ABC-SBAR" training improves simulated critical patient hand-off by pediatric interns. Pediatr Emerg Care 2012; 28: 538-43.

Newborn Life Support Course Manual 5th Edition. 2021 Resuscitation Council UK. London.

Shetty P, Cohen T, Patel B, et al. The cognitive basis of effective team performance: features of failure and success in simulated cardiac resuscitation. AMIA Annu Symp Proc 2009; 599-603.

Communicating with families

In this chapter

Principles of effective family communication

Presence of parents during resuscitation

The BAPM framework for the perinatal management for extreme prematurity in the context of communication and decision making with families

Unsuccessful resuscitation

Organ donation

The learning outcomes will enable you to:

To understand the principles of effective communication with families

Introduction

Great care is needed when communicating with the families of critically ill infants. The basis of good communication is honesty and an ability to build a trusting relationship between the clinician and the family. Communication should always be clear, honest and open. Speculation and unrealistic assurances should be avoided.

It is very important to realise that the actual words spoken form only a small part of any communication, although you need to be careful with your choice of words. The majority of the impact of any message is taken from non-verbal signals such as vocal tone, pitch and rhythm, body language and facial expressions. Careful attention must be given to these non-verbal signals and any individual must prepare themselves and their demeanour before meeting the family.

It is also extremely important to have all the available medical and background information to hand and to plan what you would like to say before meeting families in these difficult situations. Communication experience is vital and trainees should be encouraged to watch senior discussions with families wherever possible.

Communication with families who are well known to the clinician, for example those who have had infants on the neonatal unit for some time, usually have the benefit of an established open and trusting relationship. Communication is particularly difficult when parents are not known to the clinician at all. In these circumstances, it is especially important to follow the simple rules below to help to build a rapport and encourage trust.

Following successful or unsuccessful resuscitation, particularly if the parents are not known to the clinician, it is important to spend time trying to understand as much as is known about the family's culture, religious beliefs, life choices and expectations, to prevent these becoming a barrier to effective communication. At the start of every conversation, it is useful to establish what the family already know or understand about the current situation. Make sure that you use the baby's name and the correct sex.

At the end of every conversation, it is important the parents understand what has been explained. It is our responsibility to explain using appropriate language and summarising can be helpful. Families must be given the opportunity to ask any questions. It is important to make sure that they are clear what will happen next and that they are offered time to be alone and to see their baby.

The standard of our communication has been shown to directly impact the parental experience. Effective communication can provide some consolation and reassurance during difficult circumstances whereas a lack of communication or poor-quality interactions may become a source of discontent; a potential cause of complaints and litigation and contribute to feelings of isolation, thereby adding to the burden of an already challenging situation.

Principles of effective communication with families

1. **Preparation**
   - Prepare yourself thoroughly with the medical background.
   - Know parents' / carers' names, baby's name and sex.
   - Take time to prepare what you are going to say.
   - Choose an appropriate and private environment.
   - Take a nurse with you, wherever possible.
   - Check appearance / tidy hair.

2. **Establish relationship / build rapport**
   - Establish the relationship to the child of the individuals you are talking to and establish how they would like to be addressed. Try to see parents together.
   - Introduce yourself and any other staff members present.
   - Shake hands, if culturally appropriate.

3. **Non-verbal communication**
   - Sit or position yourself next to the parents so you are on the same level.
   - Maintain eye contact.

4. **Content**
   - Briefly establish what they know and use this as the basis for ongoing communication.
   - Try to use a tone of voice and non-verbal behaviour that supports what you are saying.
   - Use simple words, avoid medical jargon wherever possible.
   - Be realistic on possible outcomes.
   - If doubt exists, be honest and do not guess.
   - Provide as much relevant information as you can about what has happened and what you expect to happen next but pace this appropriately and be aware that the family are unlikely to retain large amounts of information.
   - Consider using headlines to get your main points across, aim for clarity.

5. **Offer time for questions**

6. **Summarise**
   - If possible, provide a record of the discussion.

7. **Documentation**
   - Document a summary of the main points and share these with the team.

8. **Follow up**
   - If possible, return after a period of time to confirm understanding and answer any further questions.

Presence of parents during resuscitation

Parents of sick or premature infants on the neonatal unit may be used to being present during medical procedures and may wish to be present during resuscitation of their baby. Many parents find that witnessing that everything possible was attempted during the resuscitation of their baby provides them some comfort afterwards. Families who are present at a child's death have been shown to have less anxiety, depression and better adjustment when assessed several months later.

Parents should be offered the opportunity where possible to be present during resuscitation. If they do stay, a dedicated team member must remain with them to explain the events in a sympathetic way and to ensure parents allow the team to proceed with the resuscitation unhindered. Whenever possible, physical contact with the infant should be allowed.

When to stop resuscitation

Failure to achieve return of spontaneous circulation in newborn infants after 10–20 min of intensive resuscitation is associated with a high risk of mortality and a high-risk of moderate to severe neurodevelopmental impairment among survivors. However, there is no evidence that any specific duration of resuscitation consistently predicts mortality or moderate to severe neurodevelopmental impairment. If a newborn infant requires ongoing cardiopulmonary resuscitation (CPR) after birth despite completing all the recommended steps of resuscitation and excluding reversible causes, we suggest initiating discussion of discontinuing resuscitative efforts with the clinical team and family. A reasonable timeframe to consider this change in goals of care is around 20 min after birth. The intricate nature of this decision highlights the need for input from senior members of the neonatal team. Stopping resuscitation is discussed in Chapter 2.

Antenatal counselling for extremely preterm birth

The 2019 BAPM Framework for Perinatal Management of Extreme Preterm Birth before 27 weeks of gestation emphasises that the management of birth and the immediate neonatal period should reflect the wishes and values of parents. This is discussed in Chapter 3. Decision making should involve a step wise approach involving three key stages:

1. An assessment of risk for the baby, incorporating gestational age and factors affecting fetal and maternal health
2. Counselling parents and involving them in decision-making
3. Agreeing and communicating a management plan.

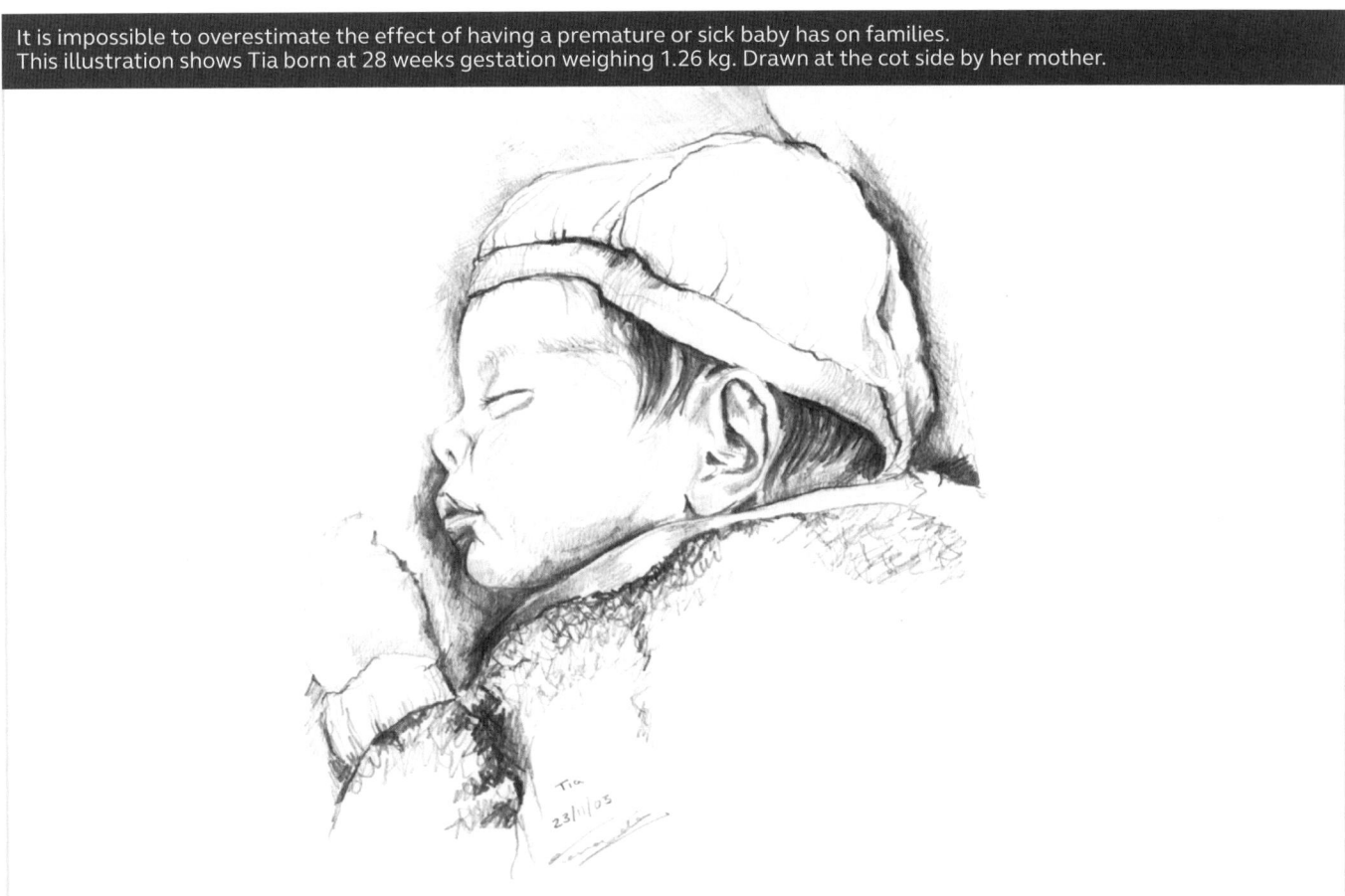

It is impossible to overestimate the effect of having a premature or sick baby has on families. This illustration shows Tia born at 28 weeks gestation weighing 1.26 kg. Drawn at the cot side by her mother.

The assessed risk category, including the associated uncertainty, must be conveyed sympathetically and with clarity. The hopes and expectations of parents should be discussed with honesty and compassion. Clear and balanced information must be provided and time for questions and clarification is essential. If survival focused care is planned, parents should be offered the chance to visit the neonatal unit, if time allows. Where a palliative approach is appropriate, the practicalities of this process must be sensitively explored to help parents prepare for possible outcomes after birth.

Unsuccessful resuscitation

Communicating the outcome following an unsuccessful resuscitation is extremely difficult. In addition, to the principles of effective communication described above, the following points also require consideration:

It is essential to confirm that you are speaking to the correct parents and establish their relationship to the baby:

- Explain with clarity that the child is dead – the words 'dead', 'died' or 'death' need to be used early in the conversation. Avoid euphemistic terms.
- Information should be given with empathy, compassion and sympathy recognising the emotional impact on the parents.
- Details of the circumstances of the death should be given clearly.
- The parents should be encouraged to see and stay with their child following the death and given the opportunity to touch and hold their child.
- Explain what will happen next.
- Ensure hand/footprints/lock of hair/photographs/name tags and other mementos are kept for parents according to local practice and parental wishes.
- Make an appointment for follow up discussion and information sharing.
- Signpost relevant support organisations/personnel.

Discussion about a post-mortem should be conducted at a suitable time and appropriate consent taken. The necessity of a post-mortem examination in the case of an unexpected death should be explored. Neonatal post-mortems should be undertaken by a perinatal pathologist. Local services vary widely but the expected time it takes for an infant to be returned for funeral arrangements must be made clear to parents. Parents often find it helpful to know about practical issues, such as how their baby will be transported to and from the pathologist. Some families with specific religious beliefs may wish to have a burial very soon after death.

If the cause of death is not known or is during or shortly following an operation, no death certificate should be issued and the case must be discussed with the Coroner, or Procurator Fiscal in Scotland, who may decide to undertake a post-mortem. Local Coroner requirements vary widely. Some regions require all child deaths to be discussed with the Coroner's office prior to certification of death. The infant's general practitioner, health visitor, local paediatrician, if applicable and other health professionals e.g. obstetrician, midwife, social worker will also need to be informed of the death.

A child death review is mandated for all children, including any live-born baby. This process incorporates a child death review meeting; an independent review by a multi-agency panel and the allocation of a key worker to provide support to the family. The review process is designed to help families to understand what has happened and to investigate whether there are any lessons to be learned.

Organ donation

If considering withdrawal of life sustaining treatment in term infants, the possibility for organ donation may be explored. If death is to be confirmed by neurological criteria then solid organ donation with the potential to save the lives of nine other children/babies is feasible and hence the wishes of the family should be sought. The donation of hepatocytes, for example, can be facilitated following cardiac death when brain stem testing is not possible or appropriate. Conversations with the family should be collaborative and the presence of a specialist nurse for organ donation is considered best practice. Prior to discussion with the family, a telephone call to the NHSBT Organ Donation Hub in the UK (available 24 h a day) ensures that accurate information can be provided about the potential for donation. Tissue donation is an additional option within 24 h of death and can provide life enhancing help to others.

06: Summary learning

Good communication with families is built on honesty and trust.

It is essential to prepare yourself and be aware of relevant medical information.

Careful attention must be paid to non-verbal communication and the utmost sensitivity and respect for families must be shown at all times.

My key take-home messages from this chapter are:

Further reading

Academy of Medical Royal Colleges. A code of practice for the diagnosis and confirmation of death. London. 2008.

British Association of Perinatal Medicine. Perinatal management of extreme preterm birth before 27 weeks gestation: a framework for practice. October 2019.

BLISS. Making critical care decisions for your baby. 2011 www.bliss.org.uk.

BMA Medical Ethics Committee. Organ donation in the 21st Century: Time for a Consolidated Approach. BMA Publications, London. 2000.

Boss RD, Lemmon RM, Arnold RM and Donohue PM. Communicating prognosis with parents of critically ill infants: direct observation of clinical behaviours. Journal of Perinatology 2017; 37: 1224-1229.

Brierly J. Neonatal organ donation: Has the time come? Arch Dis Child Fetal Neonatal ed 2011; 96: F80-3.

British Paediatric Association. Diagnosis of brain-stem death in infants and children. In: Proceedings of the Conference of Medical Royal Colleges and their Faculties in the United Kingdom. London, 1991.

Fawke J, Tinnion RJ, Monnelly V, Ainsworth SB, Cusack J, Wyllie J. How does the BAPM Framework for Practice on Perinatal Management of Extreme Preterm Birth Before 27 Weeks of Gestation impact delivery of Newborn Life Support? A Resuscitation Council UK response. Arch Dis Child Fetal Neonatal Ed. 2020 Nov;105(6):672-674. doi: 10.1136/archdischild-2020-318927. Epub 2020 Apr 9. PMID: 32273302.

Hawkins KC, Scales A, Murphy P, et al. Current status of paediatric and neonatal organ donation in the UK. Archives of Disease in Childhood 2018; 103:210-215.

HM Government. Child Death Review. Statutory and Operational Guidance (England). 2019.

Koneya M, Barbour A. Louder Than Words. (Interpersonal communication theories). Merrill Political Science C.E. Merrill Publishing. Co, Columbus, OH. 1976.

Larcher V, Craig F, Bhogal K, et al. Making decisions to limit treatment in life-limiting and life-threatening conditions in children: a framework for practice. Archives of Disease in Childhood 2015; 100:s1-s23.

Orzalesi M and Aite L. Communication with parents in neonatal intensive care. 2011; 24 (S1): 135-137.

RCPCH. The diagnosis of death by neurological criteria (DNC) in infants less than two months old, 2015.

Together for short lives. A Neonatal pathway for babies with palliative care needs. 2009. www.togetherforshortlives.org.uk

Wigert H, Dellenmark Blom A and Bry K. Parents experiences of communication with neonatal intensive care unit staff: an interview study. BMC Pediatrics 2014, 14 (304): 1-8.

Pease A and Pease B. The definitive book of body language. Orion Books 2017.

Sawyer A, Ayers S, Bertullies S, Thomas M, Weeks AD, Yoxall CW, Duley L. Providing immediate neonatal care and resuscitation at birth beside the mother: parents' views, a qualitative study. BMJ open. 2015 Sep 1;5(9): e008495.

https://www.odt.nhs.uk/deceased-donation/best-practice-guidance/paediatric-care/

https://nhsbtdbe.blob.core.windows.net/umbraco-assets-corp/18842/form-for-the-diagnosis-of-death-using-neurological-criteria-long-version-u-2-m-may-2020.pdf

Advanced airway management

07

In this chapter

Airway opening manoeuvres

Using airway adjuncts – laryngeal mask, oropharyngeal airway and nasopharyngeal airways

Oxygen delivery systems

Optimising the use of a face mask to avoid mask leak

Methods of assisted ventilation

Tracheal intubation and measuring exhaled carbon dioxide

Management of the difficult airway

The learning outcomes will enable you to:

Understand the methods used to open and maintain the neonatal airway

Understand techniques used to assist ventilation in the term and preterm infant

Be aware of techniques to minimise mask leak

Know the indications and risks of tracheal intubation and how to use other airway adjuncts

Be aware of safe strategies for the management of a baby with a difficult airway

Introduction

The majority of babies requiring resuscitation will respond to basic airway opening manoeuvres and assisted ventilation. This chapter builds on the basic airway techniques covered in the NLS manual.

It is recognised that a minority of babies will benefit from more advanced airway techniques (e.g. tracheal intubation) to facilitate a safe and secure airway for effective ventilation. Providers should be aware of the relative benefits and risks involved with these techniques. The ongoing assessment and monitoring of a baby receiving advanced airway support is reliant on good team working. Occasional circumstances arise when management of the airway can prove particularly challenging. Additional skills may be required to address these in a safe and competent manner.

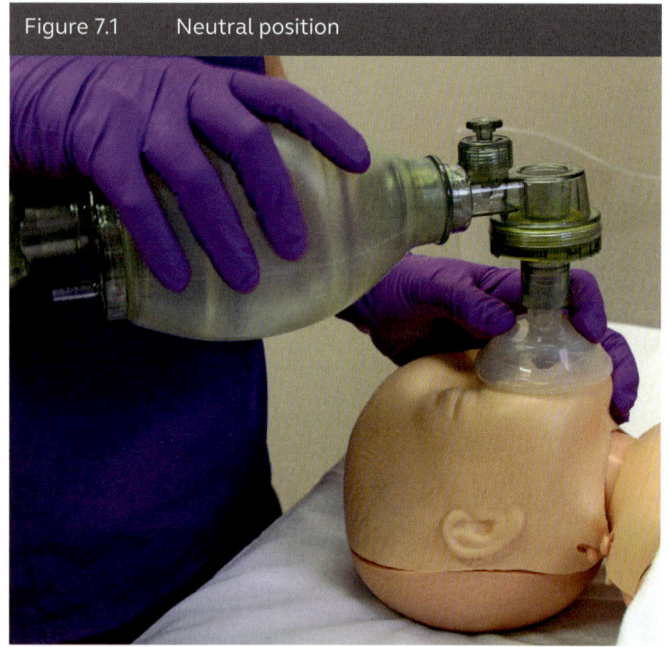

Figure 7.1 Neutral position

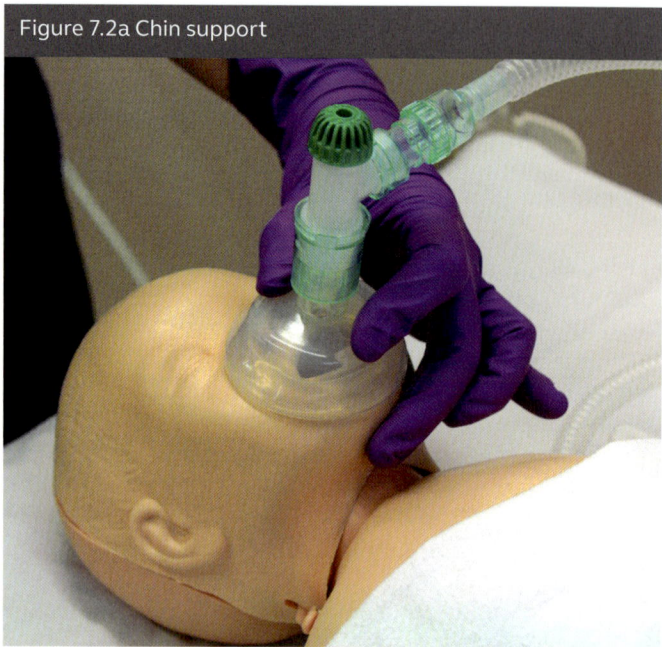

Figure 7.2a Chin support

Airway opening manoeuvres

Head position

The anatomy of the airway in newborn and young infants has a number of subtle but important differences to that in adults and older children. The tongue is relatively large and the larynx more anterior, resulting in a reduced oropharyngeal volume and potential occlusion of the upper airway. A relatively large occiput in newborn and young infants, and occasionally the head shape in preterm babies, can cause the neck to flex when the infant is placed supine. This can lead to airway compromise in an infant who has reduced muscle tone and consciousness. Airway opening manoeuvres will be required to maintain airway patency.

Neutral position

Airway obstruction can be reduced by placing the baby's head in the neutral position (Figure 7.1). The neck is neither extended nor flexed with the face parallel to the surface the baby is lying on. A 2 cm thick pad placed under the shoulders may also prove helpful in maintaining the correct position.

Chin support

Chin support is one of the most common techniques used to open the airway. In this manoeuvre, the chin is supported to pull the lower jaw forward. This widens the space at the back of the pharynx. Pressure on the soft tissues under the jaw should be avoided. Chin support can be provided whilst using a mask to deliver continuous positive airway pressure (CPAP) with or without supplemental oxygen (Figure 7.2a). Sometimes greater support of the jaw is required (Figure 7.2b).

Two-person jaw thrust

During mask ventilation in newborn infants, jaw thrust achieves a patent upper airway and reduces airway obstruction more effectively than neutral position and chin lift alone. During jaw thrust, the jaw is displaced upwards and forwards with the fingers of both hands positioned behind the angle of the jaw (Figure 7.3). This forward displacement of the mandible lifts the base of the tongue and epiglottis, actively widens the pharynx reversing the collapse of the laryngeal inlet. In infants who are either spontaneously breathing or receiving positive pressure breaths, jaw thrust has been shown to improve tidal volume and inspiratory and expiratory flow.

Suction under direct vision

Routine suctioning of the baby's mouth and nose immediately the head is delivered is not recommended. Stimulation of the pharynx may induce adduction of the vocal cords and cause profound vagal bradycardia. If there is clinical suspicion of particulate matter occluding the upper airway, give inflation breaths and consider airway suction under direct vision if airway opening manoeuvres do not result in chest movement.

The mouth and oropharynx should be visualised directly using a laryngoscope. Access to a wide bore suction catheter or Yankauer sucker will be required to remove foreign material which has the potential to occlude the upper airway.

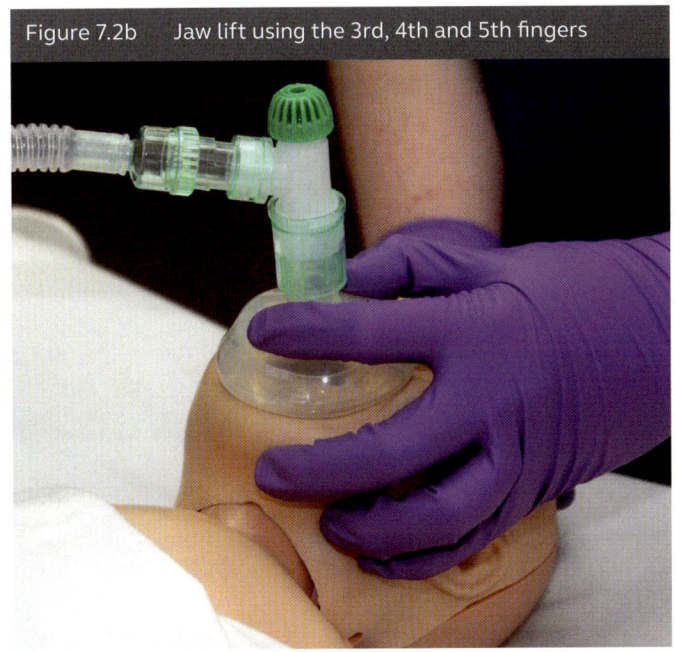

Figure 7.2b Jaw lift using the 3rd, 4th and 5th fingers

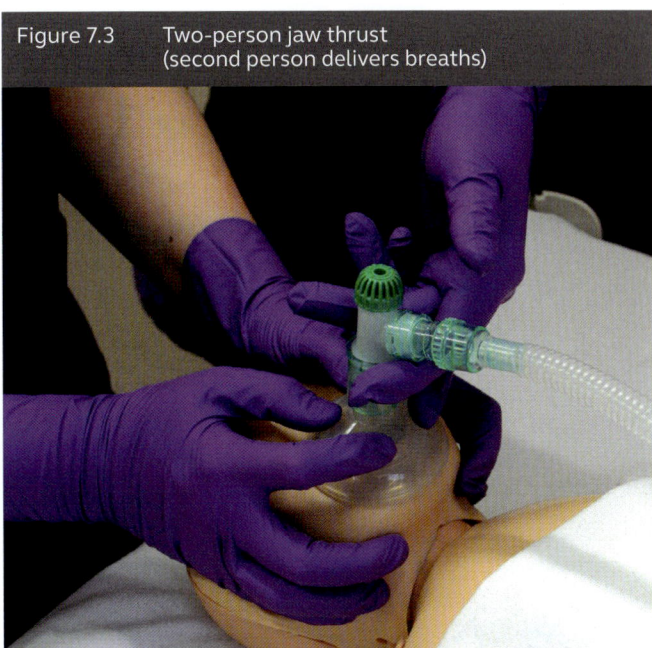

Figure 7.3 Two-person jaw thrust (second person delivers breaths)

Airway opening adjuncts

Laryngeal masks

Consider using a laryngeal mask during resuscitation of the newborn infant if face mask ventilation is unsuccessful and the chest does not move with inflation breaths. A laryngeal mask is most useful in newborn infants weighing > 2000 g or delivered after 34 weeks' gestation. It may:

- be useful if initial face mask ventilation is unsuccessful
- be considered as an alternative to tracheal intubation as a secondary airway for resuscitation
- be a useful adjunct in managing a difficult airway.

There is limited evidence evaluating its use for newborn infants weighing < 2000 g or delivered < 34 weeks' gestation and no evidence for those infants receiving compressions or in the setting of meconium-stained amniotic fluid or for the administration of emergency intra-tracheal medications.

Laryngeal mask insertion technique

- Select the correct size. Generally, a size 1 laryngeal mask is appropriate for a baby less than 5 kg and a size 1.5 for infants weighing 5–10 kg.
- Check that the laryngeal mask cuff (if present) inflates and deflates correctly. An i-gel laryngeal mask does not have an inflatable cuff (Figure 7.4).
- Lubricate the laryngeal mask with water soluble gel taking care not to occlude the lumen of the tube.
- The laryngeal mask is held so that the opening is in a forward-facing position (i.e. towards the baby's feet).
- The laryngeal mask is held 'like a pen' in the operator's dominant hand with the index finger placed just above the cuff. The device is inserted with the cuff deflated.

- A laryngoscope is recommended to support the tongue and check for particulate matter obstructing the airway.
- Position the head in a slightly extended posture and introduce the laryngeal mask into the mouth. Slide the laryngeal mask downwards and backwards along the hard palate, to reach a resting position beyond the base of the tongue. A slight resistance to any further advancement will be felt.
- Remove the laryngoscope.
- For a cuffed laryngeal mask, the cuff should be inflated using an air-filled syringe after insertion. A slight outward movement of the laryngeal mask will be observed when the cuff is inflated.
- A manual ventilation device attached to the laryngeal mask should achieve chest movement in the normal manner.
- The laryngeal mask should be secured.

If the laryngeal mask has not been successfully inserted after 30 s the baby should be ventilated using a face mask before re-attempting laryngeal mask insertion. Other options to support the airway should be considered.

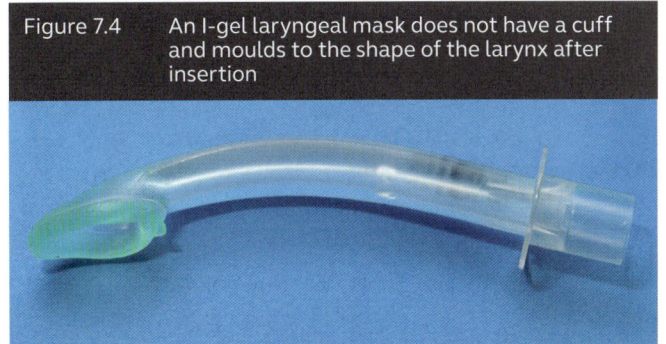

Figure 7.4 An I-gel laryngeal mask does not have a cuff and moulds to the shape of the larynx after insertion

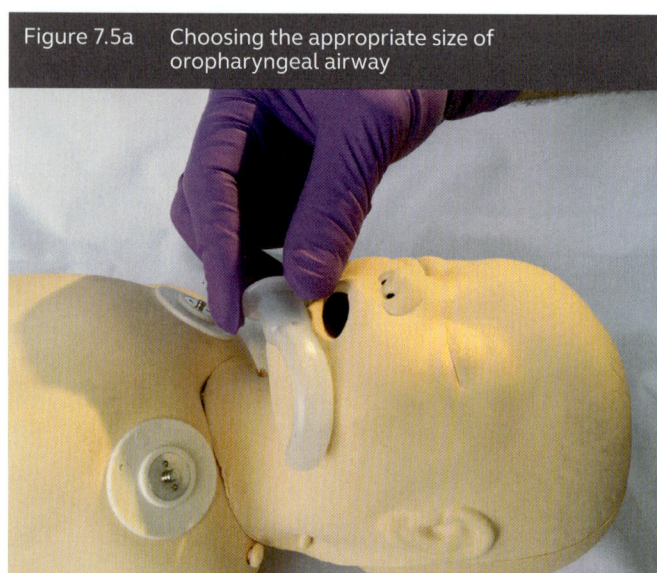

Figure 7.5a   Choosing the appropriate size of oropharyngeal airway

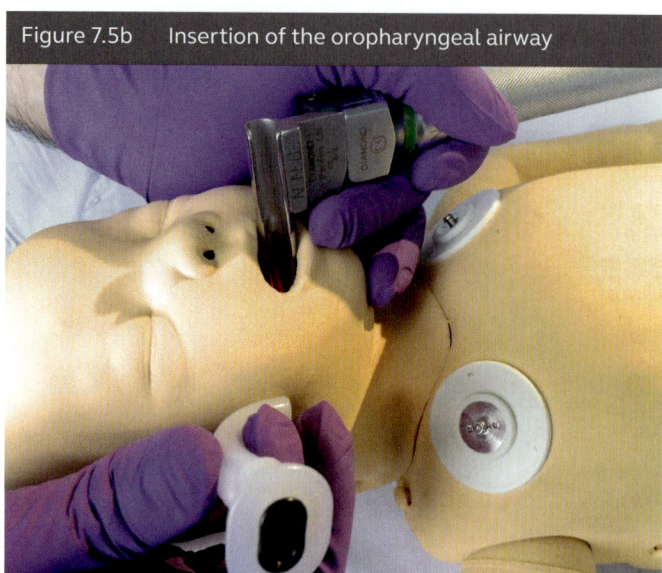

Figure 7.5b   Insertion of the oropharyngeal airway

Oropharyngeal airways

An oropharyngeal airway is a valuable adjunct. The ideal length will reach just beyond the base of the tongue helping to lift it forward out of the oropharynx. This can be particularly useful in the presence of an orofacial congenital anomaly such as micrognathia or choanal atresia. An oropharyngeal airway may also be helpful to a single operator when help is not immediately available. It is important to use the correct size as oropharyngeal airways can obstruct the airway if used incorrectly, especially in preterm babies.

A correctly sized oropharyngeal airway is measured from the middle of the lips to the angle of the jaw (Figure 7.5a). There are a range of sizes of oropharyngeal airway suitable for babies at birth. If the airway is too small it will not reach the end of the tongue and if too large may well protrude out of the mouth. An oropharyngeal airway is inserted with the curve facing downwards towards the feet by sliding the tip over the tongue, under direct vision, taking care that it does not push the tongue backwards into the mouth (Figure 7.5b). After insertion, clinical assessment should confirm that the estimated size is appropriate for that baby.

Nasopharyngeal airways

Insertion of a nasopharyngeal airway is designed to open the channel between the nostril and the nasopharynx. As most newborns are nasal breathers this technique is particularly effective in this age group. The nasopharyngeal airway is better tolerated by the conscious infant than an oropharyngeal airway. The technique is most commonly used to support an infant who has partial upper airway obstruction with patent nasal passageways and an adequate respiratory drive. This includes babies with congenital anomalies such as micrognathia and cleft lip and palate or other pathology causing restriction of nasopharyngeal or oropharyngeal spaces.

The nasopharyngeal airway is a soft flexible plastic or silicone bevelled tube. Once sited the additional flange material may be cut down and used to secure the device in the correct position. A standard tracheal tube can also be used as a neonatal nasopharyngeal airway (Figure 7.6). The appropriate size tube can be estimated by visually matching its diameter against the internal diameter of the nostril. The length can be estimated from the distance between the tip of the nose and tragus of the ear.

The nasopharyngeal airway should be lubricated and introduced into the nostril with a gentle rotating motion passing the airway directly backwards and posteriorly along the floor of the nostril. The length of the airway should be confirmed by direct vision with a laryngoscope, observing that the tip of the device appears in view at the top of the oropharynx. A correctly sized tube should fit snugly in the nostril without causing blanching of the nares.

This device is not suitable for infants with obstruction to the choanal space, significant coagulopathy or if there are copious or tenacious secretions.

Oxygen delivery systems

Oxygen mask

A simple oxygen mask may be used to provide supplemental oxygen in a spontaneously breathing infant. This can achieve a maximum oxygen concentration of approximately 60%; adding a rebreathing bag can increase this to almost 100%. The high flow rates of cold, dry gases are poorly tolerated in neonates. Other than short term intervention, alternative oxygen delivery systems may be preferable if more prolonged supplementation is required.

Nasal cannula

This may be useful in stable babies who are breathing spontaneously. Oxygen delivery via cannula (or 'prongs') is dependent on oxygen flow and nasal resistance so it is not suitable during resuscitation or when a high oxygen concentration is required. Low flow systems can be tolerated up to a maximum of 1 L min^{-1}. High-flow nasal cannula systems deliver warmed and humidified gases; flow is set at up to 8 L min^{-1}. This continuous flow of gas can provide higher oxygen concentrations with additional respiratory support via a 'washout' effect of the nasopharynx.

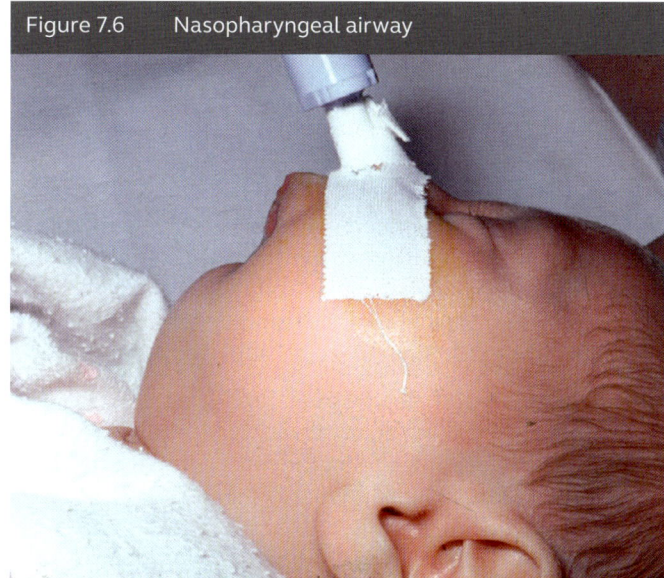

Figure 7.6 Nasopharyngeal airway

Head box oxygen

This method is more commonly used in larger babies in the paediatric setting but may be used in small infants. It permits reliable measurement and control of the inspired oxygen level, as well as allowing warming and humidification of the delivered oxygen. However, the oxygen level falls rapidly when the lid is removed from the headbox to undertake care procedures or a full assessment of the infant's clinical condition. Rapid access to the infant's head can be difficult and therefore headbox delivery is not appropriate during resuscitation.

Face mask ventilation

Face masks are manufactured in a variety of shapes and sizes (Figure 7.7). The selected mask should conform to the baby's facial contours to form a virtually airtight seal. The mask should cover the nose and mouth without extending over the edge of the jaw or encroaching on the orbits, Table 7.1 gives suggested mask sizes. Round silicone masks are often easier to use. Providing even pressure is applied to the top surface of the mask, the soft flange will deform to the contours of the face minimising mask leak; which is a common reason for failure of mask ventilation in newborn resuscitation.

Table 7.1 Estimating face mask size by gestation and/or birthweight

Gestation	Mask size	Weight
23 weeks	35 mm	< 1000 g
24 weeks		
25 weeks		
26 weeks		
27 weeks	35 or 42 mm	1000–1249 g
28 weeks		
29 weeks	42 mm	1250–2000 g
30 weeks		
31 weeks		
32 weeks		
33–34 weeks	42 or 50 mm	2000–2499 g
35–36 weeks		
37 weeks	50 mm	< 3000 g
Term IUGR / 38 weeks	50 or 60 mm	> 3000 g
> 39 weeks / LGA	60 mm	> 3500 g

Note: 50 mm = size 0/0 or size 0 and a 60 mm = size 0/1 or size 1, dependent on manufacturer

What's the evidence?

Facemask ventilation is used for infants who are apnoeic or have inadequate breathing. At birth it may facilitate the clearance of lung fluid, establish and maintain a resting lung volume and thereby ensure aeration.

Good mask ventilation technique requires that you have an open airway, a well-fitting mask, a suitable ventilation device and an effective technique for creating a virtually air-tight seal between the mask and face. This seemingly simple technique is difficult to master and has been the subject of numerous manikin and infant studies.

Studies involving doctors, nurses and midwives of all grades have shown significant mask leaks are common

Figure 7.7 A selection of suitable masks

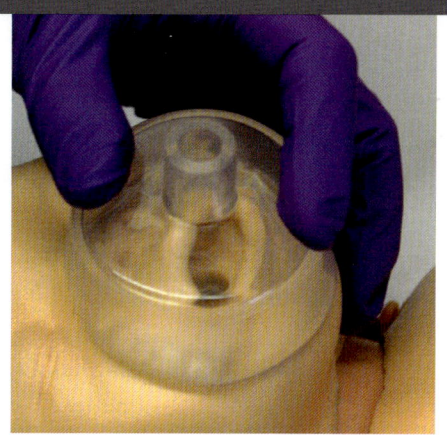
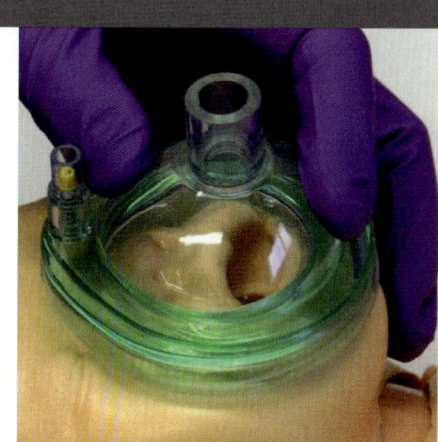

during face mask ventilation. Whilst the optimal amount of mask leak is unknown, large leaks are associated with reduced tidal volume and consequently poor ventilation. With little or no leak excessive tidal volume and over ventilation may occur. Crucially it has been demonstrated that mask leak can vary on an almost breath to breath basis resulting in the potential for both dangerously low and excessively high tidal volumes. This can be further compounded by airway obstruction. Both mask leak and airway obstruction are common issues affecting preterm airway management.

Reducing variation in leak allows for more consistent ventilation. This facilitates more accurate assessment of chest movement and appropriate adjustment of ventilation settings.

Research has identified that face mask ventilation technique is far more important than equipment used. Direct feedback systems have been shown to improve resuscitator performance and clinical outcomes in the delivery room.

ARNI course face mask ventilation station

A system has been specifically designed for this course to enable candidates to benefit from objective and immediate feedback on their mask ventilation technique.

Similar systems have been used in the research evaluating masks, ventilation devices, resuscitator techniques, and effectiveness of training; and continue to be used to identify knowledge gaps.

Simple steps and minor changes can improve the efficiency of face mask ventilation and this station uses computer feedback to improve individual candidate's performance. Studies have defined the '3 key ways to reduce mask leak'; to reproducibly achieve a virtually air-tight seal:

1. rolling the mask onto the face ('align, roll, check') (Figure 7.8) for a correct mask position
2. balancing the pressure exerted on the mask by the finger and thumb
3. lifting or pulling the jaw upwards into the mask.

These 3 steps used correctly can ensure that an effective mask seal is created; they can be applied to any mask design, term and preterm resuscitation and all single resuscitator mask holds or two-person techniques. These steps can be used to quickly identify and correct sources of mask leak (Figure 7.8 and Appendix B).

Many candidates will have identified a mask hold that works for them, potentially over years of clinical practice and will already have a good mask ventilation technique. However, this is not universal and for every candidate there are learning opportunities and the possibility to further enhance their technique using the above themes.

The ARNI course face mask ventilation station teaches techniques that work for the majority (Figure 7.9). The 'Two-point top hold' is the most widely tested of the mask holds. It has been shown to be the most effective for the majority of resuscitators and mask designs.

Positioning the mask onto the baby's face

A technique of rolling the mask from the chin towards the bridge of the nose achieves decreased mask leak by ensuring consistent and correct positioning of the mask (Figures 7.10a and b). The operator's thumb and index fingers should be placed on the top surface of the mask with the third, fourth and fifth fingers aligned along the mandibular ridge providing jaw lift. Care should be taken to avoid pressure on the soft tissues under the chin as this may close the airway. The thenar eminence of the hand may be placed lightly on the baby's forehead to stabilise the 'neutral' position and allow for fine adjustment of flexion or extension to achieve optimal airway opening.

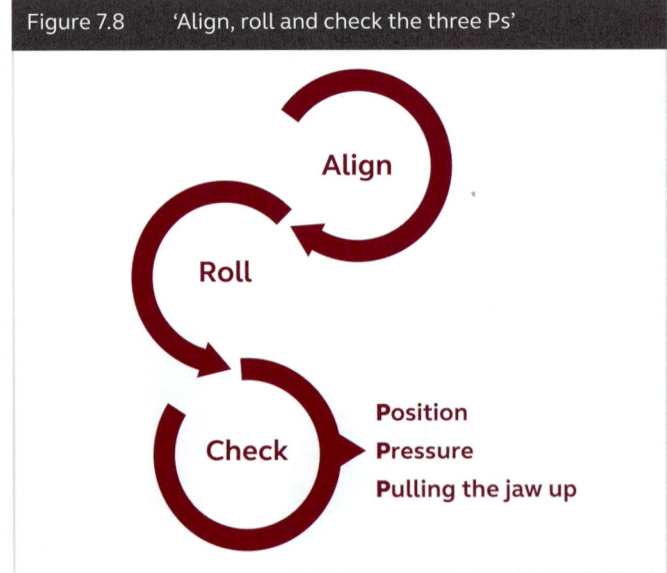

Figure 7.8   'Align, roll and check the three Ps'

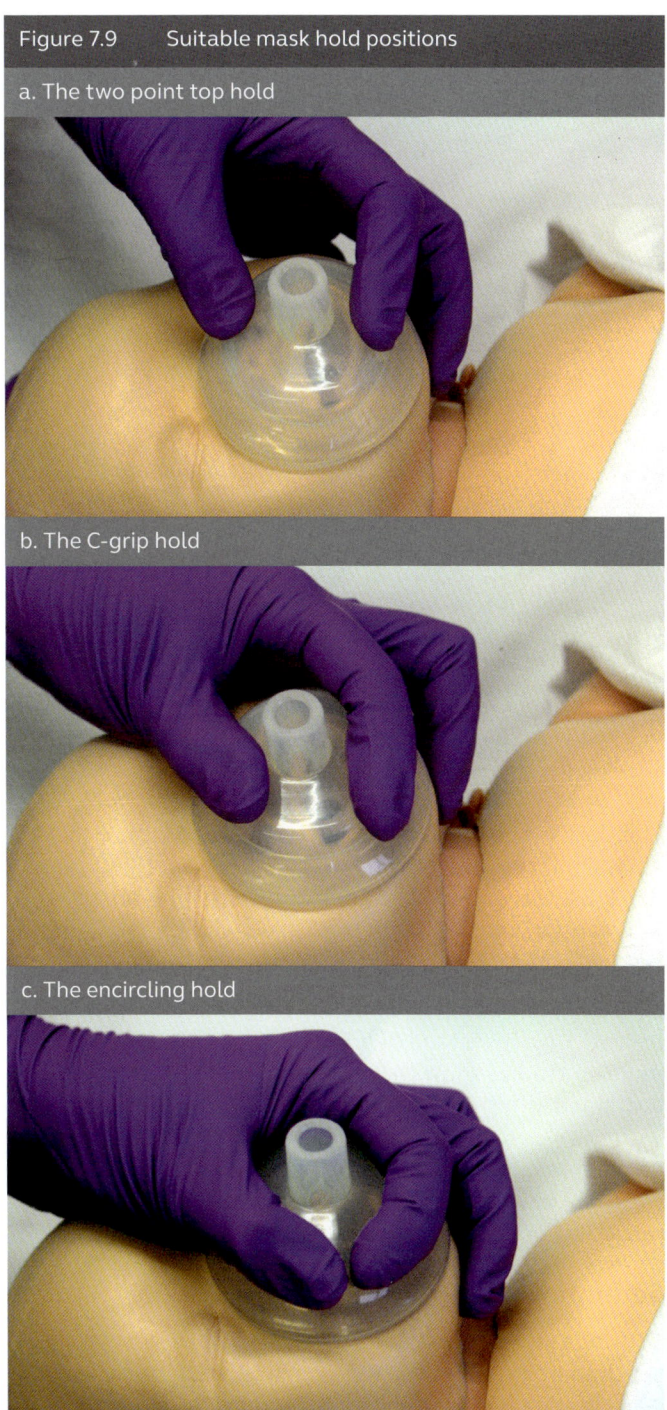

Figure 7.9 Suitable mask hold positions

a. The two point top hold

b. The C-grip hold

c. The encircling hold

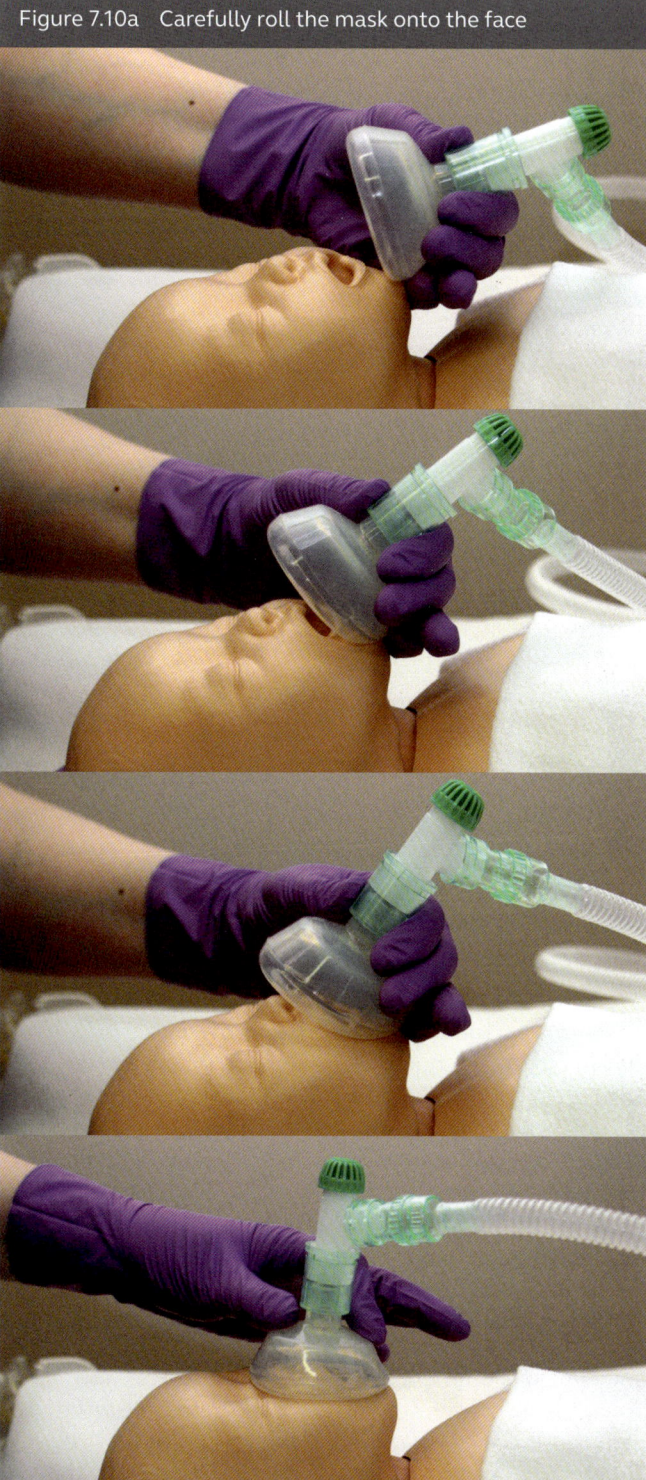

Figure 7.10a Carefully roll the mask onto the face

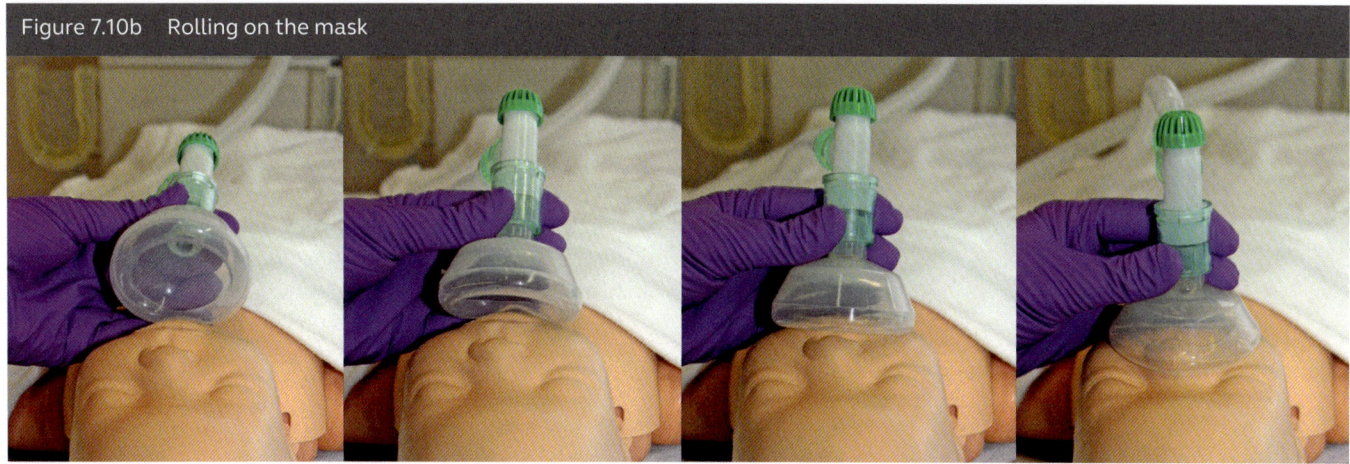

Figure 7.10b Rolling on the mask

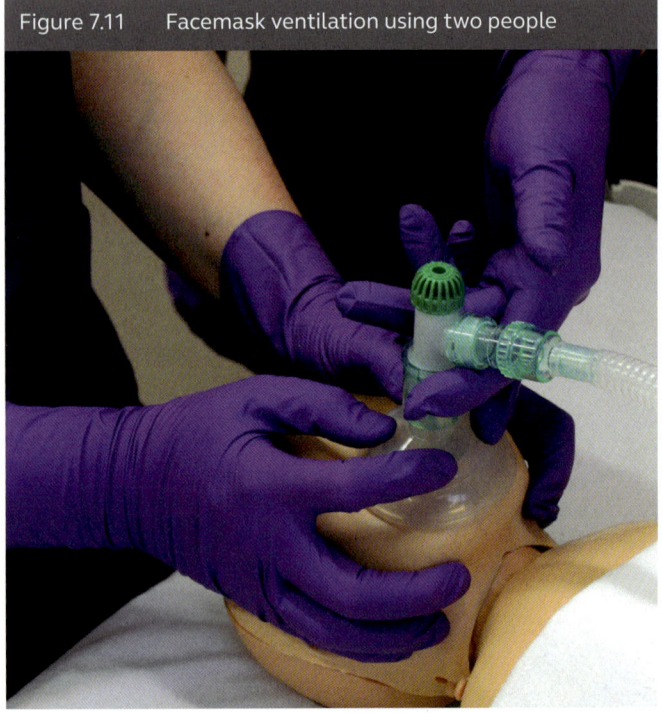

Figure 7.11   Facemask ventilation using two people

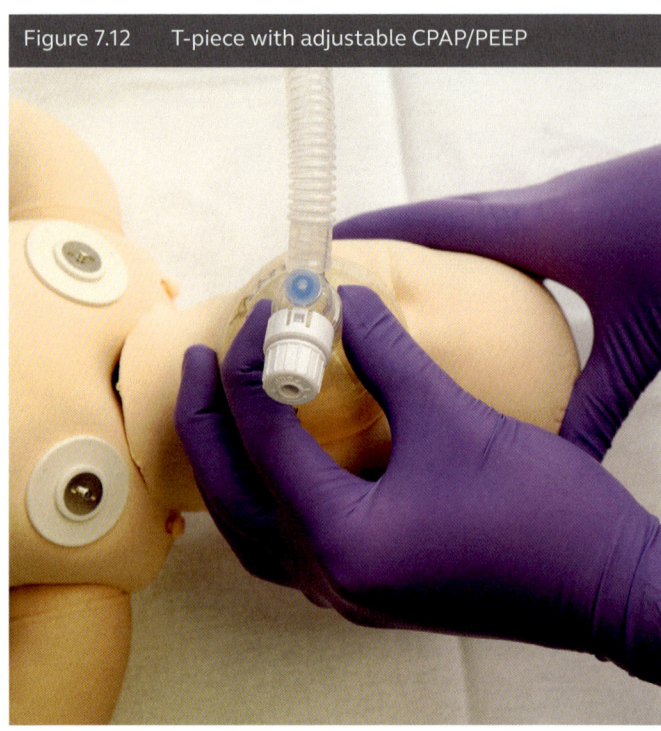

Figure 7.12   T-piece with adjustable CPAP/PEEP

Face mask ventilation using two people

It may be difficult for a single operator to achieve effective mask ventilation. Mask leak and delivery of appropriate tidal volumes are improved using a two-person technique. One person maintains airway position and mask seal whilst the second person provides ventilation. Both people can see if the chest is rising and should make appropriate adjustments until this occurs (Figure 7.11).

Methods of assisted ventilation

Delivery of effective positive pressure ventilation is vital to successful neonatal resuscitation. Current guidelines recommend the use of three devices: the T-piece resuscitator, self-inflating bag, and flow-inflating bag. These devices may be attached to a face mask or directly to a laryngeal mask or tracheal tube, once these are in place.

T-piece resuscitator

A T-piece device requires a pressurised gas supply. A continuous gas flow of up to 8 L min^{-1} is commonly used but should be guided by device manufacturer's recommendations. Regulating the flow of gas through the T-piece alters the pressure that can be delivered. The maximum pressure is controlled by the adjustable pressure blow-off valve within the device and the positive end expiratory pressure (PEEP) is usually adjusted by a screw device in the circuit itself. Occlusion of the valve (Figure 7.12) delivers the peak inspiratory pressure (PIP).

The user should be aware that changes in gas flow may have significant effects on PIP and PEEP. A self-inflating bag should always be available in case there is an interruption in gas supply. The T-piece device should never be connected directly to the wall gas supply.

There is limited clinical evidence of low certainty that using a T-piece instead of a SIB reduces BPD. However, manikin studies show that target inflation pressures, sustained inflation breaths and PEEP are easier to deliver with the T-piece. Tidal volumes delivered are smaller and less variable. Care should be taken to ensure that the PEEP valve is not inadvertently tightened during the resuscitation.

Self-inflating bag with mask ventilation

Self-Inflating bag (also known as bag valve mask) ventilation describes the use of a face mask and a self-inflating bag system with or without an oxygen reservoir attached that delivers positive pressure ventilation without re-breathing of exhaled respiratory gases. A 'blow off' valve provides a pressure limit in the circuit and this should always be tested prior to use.

Self-inflating bags are available in a range of sizes, the 500 mL version is the most commonly used in neonatal resuscitation. Squeezing the bag provides forward flow of gas through a one-way valve and providing there is adequate mask seal, lung inflation will be achieved. Once inspiratory flow is terminated, expiratory recoil of the chest occurs and gas is passively exhaled. The elastic properties of the self-inflating bag allow refilling in anticipation of the next actively delivered inspiratory breath. The device operates effectively without a supplementary gas flow. However, oxygen enrichment can be achieved up to approximately 50% by attaching a high flow of oxygen to the port on the base of the bag and to over 90% using a reservoir bag.

Care should be taken to avoid delivery of excessive tidal volumes or undue force exerted downwards onto the baby's face. Vigorous and uncontrolled squeezing of the bag can generate a high flow of gas and pressures of 60–80 cm H_2O can be produced; whilst there is a pressure limiting blow off valve this is flow sensitive and may not prevent excessive pressure. A gas flow of 10 L min^{-1} is commonly used if supplemental oxygen is required.. Continuous monitoring of the heart rate and oxygen saturations should be undertaken as soon as practical. Self inflating bags should not be used to deliver oxygen in spontaneously breathing infants as they may not be able to generate sufficient pressures to overcome the valve.

Flow inflating bag mask circuits

This equipment is generally used by anaesthetic staff and is not commonly used on neonatal units. The circuit is flow dependent with no 'blow off' valve. To achieve ventilation the open end of the bag is occluded by the operator and the bag is squeezed. In inexperienced hands a flow inflating bag can deliver excessive pressures or tidal volumes.

Tracheal intubation

Neonatal tracheal intubation, like all practical skills, is acquired by appropriate training initially using manikins, before progressing to supervised experience in real situations.

Intubation can be more difficult in infants than older children or adults. Most newborns will respond to mask ventilation, and providing this is effective, there should be no need to perform tracheal intubation until experienced personnel are available. Remember laryngeal mask insertion may also be an option. An understanding of the indications for intubation, anatomical considerations and equipment required for this technique are helpful.

Tracheal intubation is a 'gold standard' method to achieve and maintain a secure airway and in some circumstances, is the technique of choice. Intubation may be useful in a prolonged resuscitation and in preterm infants for the administration of surfactant. Early and elective intubation of babies with an antenatal diagnosis of congenital diaphragmatic hernia is recommended as this minimises air insufflation of the stomach or bowel contained within the chest. Intubation may be helpful if the airway is blocked with inhaled material.

Indications for neonatal tracheal intubation

- Prolonged apnoea
- Ineffective mask ventilation
- During a prolonged resuscitation
- Administration of surfactant
- A period of mechanical ventilation support is anticipated (e.g. respiratory distress syndrome, surgery)
- Severe anatomical or functional upper airway obstruction
- When gastric insufflation would compromise ventilation (e.g. congenital diaphragmatic hernia)
- To provide tracheal or bronchial suctioning
- If high pressures are required to maintain adequate oxygenation
- Instability or high probability that problems may occur before or during a transport episode
- High or increasing oxygen requirements on non-invasive respiratory support.

Anatomical considerations

Babies have a relatively large tongue, a high anterior larynx and a narrow 'U' shaped epiglottis. The narrowest part of the airway is at the cricoid ring.

Equipment

Tracheal tubes

Uncuffed tracheal tubes are used in neonatal intubation because of the unique anatomical shape of the airway. Tracheal tubes are sized by their internal diameter in millimetres. Manufacturing differences can mean that tracheal tubes with the same internal diameter can have different external diameters.

Laryngoscope

This consists of a handle usually containing batteries, a light source and a blade. Straight blades (size 00, 0 and 1) are usually preferred for intubation of the newborn. The straight blade is designed to hold the tongue out of the way and to lift the epiglottis under the tip of the blade so that the vocal cords can be seen.

Indirect laryngoscopy using video laryngoscopic devices may be helpful in ensuring correct catheter position with less invasive surfactant administration (LISA) or in assisting in the management of the difficult tracheal intubation. A video attached to these devices also has a valuable role in teaching intubation skills.

Intubation technique

Ideally the baby should have heart rate and oxygen saturation monitoring in place; consider aspirating the stomach before attempting intubation. Prior to intubation the infant should be ventilated using mask ventilation while the equipment is checked. The following equipment may be needed:

- intubation medications (if required) as per local protocol
- T-piece device or self-inflating bag with pressure release valve
- appropriately sized face mask
- blended oxygen / air supply
- laryngoscope handles and blades in a range of sizes e.g. 00, 0, 1
- uncuffed tracheal tubes in a range of sizes e.g. 2.5, 3.0, 3.5, 4.0 mm
- stylet (according to local protocol)
- Magill's forceps (for nasal intubation)
- tapes or bespoke attachments to secure the tracheal tube
- suction apparatus and catheters
- end-tidal carbon dioxide monitoring/colour change capnography.

Sterility of equipment should be maintained until used. The infant's head is placed in a slightly extended position, remembering that the commonest error in tracheal intubation is over-extension of the neck.

The laryngoscope blade is gently advanced inside the mouth. The tongue and epiglottis are pulled forward by gently lifting the blade. If the vocal cords and epiglottis do not come into view the laryngoscope should be pulled back gradually until they can be seen, to avoid intubation of the oesophagus. Adjunct techniques such as centrally applied cricoid pressure, use of a stylet or a longer laryngoscope blade may be helpful. The tracheal tube should be passed through the vocal cords under direct vision and held firmly in position whilst the laryngoscope blade is gently removed.

A 3.5 mm tube is suitable for a term baby, though it is wise to have half a size larger and smaller to hand. It is important to have a snug fit to reduce the leak of gas between the tube and the tracheal wall. The tube should be able to slide into the trachea with minimal resistance and come to lie with the tip above the carina. Suggested tracheal tube lengths are shown in Table 7.2. Some tracheal tubes have black markings at the tip indicating the length that the tube needs to pass through the vocal cords to rest in the mid-trachea. If a stylet is used, care should be taken to ensure that it is fixed so that the tip does not protrude beyond the end of the tracheal tube as this may cause trauma to the trachea.

Attempts to intubate should take no longer than 30 s. If tracheal intubation is not successful, or if there is desaturation or bradycardia, mask ventilation should be provided. A maximum of two attempts per person is generally recommended and no more than four attempts in total. This reduces the risk of upper airway trauma, oedema and bleeding and highlights to the team that an alternative strategy may need to be deployed. Clear guidelines should ensure that all members of the team are empowered to call for an alternative strategy to be deployed and for senior assistance to be summoned.

Intubation with sedation and muscle relaxation

Intubation causes physiological instability and is distressing and painful. The effects can be reduced by premedication with sedation and muscle relaxation. At delivery or in potentially life-threatening situations, intubation without sedation is appropriate.

In controlled situations the decision to use premedication will depend on the experience and training of the operator and on local policy. Since intubation of an active baby is more difficult, premedication is particularly relevant to more mature babies.

One accepted regime for premedication prior to tracheal intubation would comprise:

- atropine 10–30 microgram kg^{-1} IV (maximum 100 micrograms)
- morphine 100 microgram kg^{-1} IV (allow 3–5 min to take effect)
- suxamethonium 1.5–3.0 microgram kg^{-1} given as a slow IV bolus 3 to 5 min after morphine administration.

Table 7.2 A guide to tracheal tubes sizes and approximate lengths

Gestational age	Birth weight	Size TT ID	Length at lips	Length at nose
25 weeks	650 g	2.5 mm	6.0 cm	7.0 cm
28 weeks	1200 g	2.5 mm	7.0 cm	8.0 cm
31 weeks	1600 g	2.5 / 3.0 mm	7.5 cm	8.5 cm
34 weeks	2400 g	3.0 mm	8.0 cm	9.0 cm
37 weeks	3000 g	3.0 mm	9.0 cm	10.5 cm
40 weeks	3500 g	3.5 mm	9.5 cm	11.0 cm

Fentanyl 2 microgram kg^{-1} IV over 30 s may be used as an alternative to morphine and has a faster onset of action. Fentanyl should be given slowly, as rapid administration has been associated with chest wall spasm.

Verification of tracheal tube placement

The position of the tube should be checked by several methods as no single method is completely reliable.
- direct visualization of the tube passing through the vocal cords
- seeing moisture in the tracheal tube during expiration
- detection of exhaled carbon dioxide by capnography.
- observed symmetrical rise of the chest
- auscultation of air entry on both sides of the chest
- positive response in vital signs: heart rate, oxygen saturations
- radiological (tube tip positioned at the level of T2–T3).

End-tidal CO_2 detection

Detection of exhaled CO_2 confirms tracheal intubation in neonates with a cardiac output more rapidly and more accurately than clinical assessment alone. It will not distinguish between a correctly placed tracheal tube in the trachea and a long tracheal tube with the tip in the right main bronchus. False negative readings may occur in very low birth weight neonates and in infants during cardiac arrest (in these cases a brief period of chest compressions may bring about a colour change as more CO_2 is delivered to the lungs). False positives may occur with colorimetric devices contaminated with adrenaline, surfactant, atropine or water.

End-tidal CO_2 detection should be used in neonatal intubation; alternatively continuous waveform capnography is increasingly used in some neonatal settings and can indicate if a tracheal tube has become blocked or dislodged.

Once the tracheal tube position has been confirmed, it is important to set up the ventilator. Typical starting settings using time cycled, pressure-controlled ventilation for a baby would be a PIP of around 18 cm H_2O, a PEEP of 4–5 cm H_2O, a rate of 40 breaths per minute and an inspiratory time of 0.3–0.4 s. If using volume-controlled ventilation tidal volumes of 4 to 8 mL kg^{-1} are commonly used.

Management of the difficult airway – maintaining a safe approach

The majority of infants requiring resuscitation at birth will respond to basic airway manoeuvres and mask ventilation, providing this is performed correctly, with an open airway and good mask seal. For some infants other airway adjuncts (e.g. laryngeal mask, oro- or naso- pharyngeal airway) may be helpful, others may benefit from intubation.

Once this technique is mastered by the practitioner, this is usually a relatively straightforward procedure. There are, however, a minority of babies who have a 'difficult airway' and in these circumstances achieving and maintaining a safe airway can be extremely challenging. A difficult airway can occur in babies with craniofacial abnormalities such as Pierre Robin sequence (cleft palate and micrognathia) or Treacher Collins syndrome. Neck masses such as a cystic hygroma or teratoma may cause problems with the airway. Neuromuscular abnormalities may sometimes result in restricted neck movement making it more difficult to open the airway effectively.

The management of a baby with a difficult airway is easier if the situation has been predicted and appropriate support planned in advance. Effective antenatal screening and good communication between professionals will allow for delivery in an appropriate centre. A clearly established plan which might involve multi-disciplinary teams and specialised equipment may be required.

For a baby with an unanticipated difficult airway, it is important to have a locally agreed escalation policy. It is helpful to have an accessible resource of additional airway equipment, located in a prominent position in the department which is well known to the staff (Table 7.3). Rehearsal using 'point of care' simulation training allows teams to be well prepared and familiar with the team working skills and access to additional support which may be required.

Table 7.3 Suggested equipment for a 'difficult airway' escalation box

500 mL self-inflating bag
Soft round masks (size 1, 0, 00)
Oropharyngeal airways (ISO size 3.5, 5.0, 5.5. Previously labelled 000,00,0)
Straight blade laryngoscope (size 0, 1)
Curved blade laryngoscope (e.g. Macintosh)
Tracheal tubes (2.5, 3.0, 3.5, 4.0)
Intubation stylet
Carbon dioxide detector device
Oxygen saturation monitor and probes
Magill's forceps
Bougie
Supraglottic airway devices:
LMA (size 1, 1.5); i-gel (size 1)
Optical laryngoscopic devices: eg: Airtraq
Flexible fibreoptic bronchoscope
Rigid bronchoscope
Tracheostomy instrument set
Pulse oximetry
End-tidal CO_2 monitoring

Figure 7.13   An example of a 'difficult airway escalation policy'

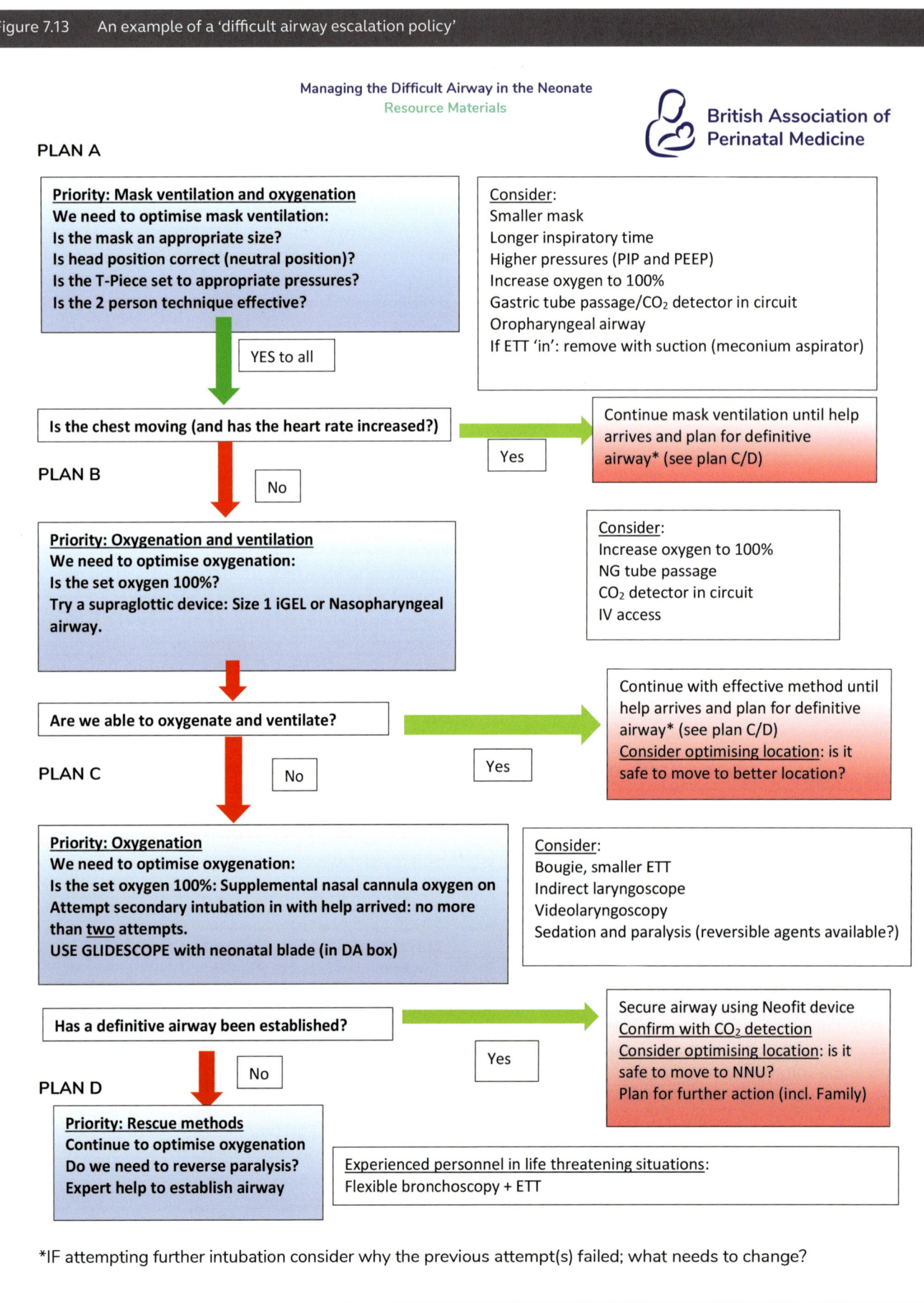

The framework illustrated in Figure 7.13 is reproduced from the British Association of Perinatal Medicine (with permission) and shows an example of a difficult airway escalation policy which can be adapted to local needs. Competent basic airway manoeuvres and mask ventilation underpin the approach to newborn resuscitation and this pathway assumes that these approaches have been unsuccessful and / or a more definitive airway management is required.

The ability to promptly recognise a situation when an airway is challenging will allow timely and appropriate recruitment of senior help. The priority to maintain oxygenation and ventilation should remain paramount. Effective team working and communication are key; it is very easy to fall into a trap of 'task fixation', resulting in repeated attempts to intubate with increasing upper airway trauma, hypoxaemia and worsening bradycardia. If tracheal intubation has failed, it is important to return quickly and safely to optimising mask ventilation using the manoeuvres previously described if at all possible. Remember the importance of correct head positioning, jaw thrust, a two-person technique and consider inserting a laryngeal mask, oropharyngeal or nasopharyngeal airway. Success in maintaining oxygenation and ventilation in this way combined with calling for senior help allows time for a carefully considered plan to manage the airway. Once help arrives, consideration may be given to re-attempting direct laryngoscopy with the help of cricoid pressure, use of an introducer or stylet, or using a longer laryngoscope blade.

'Can't intubate, can't ventilate'

The situation in which intubation has failed and the baby is unable to be ventilated using mask ventilation techniques and airway adjuncts is a frightening one which emphasizes the need for prompt recognition and an early call for help. Options in this situation include placement of a laryngeal mask, the use of a bougie or optical laryngoscope to facilitate intubation. Anaesthetic, ENT or surgical colleagues may consider the use of a flexible fibreoptic or rigid bronchoscope.

When neither tracheal intubation or ventilation are possible using any of the above techniques it is important to appreciate that rescue techniques including cutaneous tracheal puncture, cricothyroidotomy and tracheostomy may be attempted, but only by experienced and trained people in life threatening situations.

07: Summary learning

Effective management of the airway is vital.

Mask position and techniques to reduce mask leak are important.

Airway adjuncts including laryngeal masks, oropharyngeal and nasopharyngeal airways can be helpful.

Good preparation and skilled assistants make successful tracheal tube placement more likely.

Safe practice around intubation is essential; once placed a tracheal tube should be secured and checked.

A structured approach to a difficult airway can be lifesaving.

My key take-home messages from this chapter are:

Further reading

Bowman TA, Paget-Brown A, Carroll J, Gurka MJ, Kattwinkel J. Sensing and responding to compliance changes during manual ventilation using a lung model: can we teach healthcare providers to improve? J Pediatr 2012; 160(3): 372-376 e1.

Chua C, Schmoler GM, Davis P. Airway manoeuvres to achieve upper airway patency during mask ventilation in newborn infants - a historical perspective". Resuscitation 2012; 8: 411-416.

Crocker K, Black A. Assessment of the predicted difficult airway in babies and children. Anaesthesia and intensive care medicine 2009;10(4):200-205.

Difficult Airway Society (UK). Difficult Airway Society guidelines 2004 www.das.uk.com

Managing the difficult airway in the Neonate: A BAPM Framework for practice (October 2020). https://www.bapm.org/resources/199-managing-the-difficult-airway-in-the-neonate

Esmail N, Saleh M, Ali A. Laryngeal mask airway versus endotracheal intubation for Apgar score improvement in neonatal resuscitation. Egyptian J Anesthesiol 2002; 18: 115-21.

Finer NN, Rich W, Wang C, Leone T. Airway obstruction during mask ventilation of very low birth weight infants during neonatal resuscitation. Pediatrics 2009; 123: 865-869.

Haase B, Badinska AM, Koos B, et al. Do commonly available round facemasks fit near-term and term infants? Arch Dis Child Fetal Neonatal Ed 2020;105(4): F364-8.

Hawkes CP, Ryan CA, Dempsey EM. Comparison of the T-piece resuscitator with other neonatal manual ventilation devices: a qualitative review. Resuscitation 2012; 83: 797-802.

Kamlin CO, Schillerman K, Dawson JA et al. Mask versus nasal tube for stabilization of preterm infants at birth: A randomised controlled trial. Pediatrics 2013; 132(2): 1-8.

O'Donnell CPF, Davis PG, Lau R et al. Neonatal resuscitation 2: an evaluation of manual ventilation devices and facemasks. Arch Dis Child Fetal Neonatal Ed 2005; 90: F392-6.

O'Shea JE, Thio M et al. Measurements from preterm infants to guide face mask size. Measurements from preterm infants to guide face mask size. Arch Dis Child Fetal Neonatal Ed 2016;101: F294-8.

Poulton DA, Schmiilzer GM, Morley CJ, Davis PG. Assessment of chest rise during mask ventilation of preterm infants in the delivery room. Resuscitation 2011; 82: 175-9.

Schmiilzer GM, Kamlin CO, O'Donnell CPF, Dawson JA, Morley CJ, Davis PG. Assessment of tidal volume and gas leak during mask ventilation of preterm infants in the delivery room. Arch Dis Child Fetal Neonatal Ed 201 O; 95: F393-7.

Schmolzer GM, Dawson JA, Kamlin CO, O'Donnell CPF, Morley CJ, Davis PG. Airway obstruction and gas leak during mask ventilation of preterm infants in the delivery room. Arch Dis Child Fetal Neonatal Ed 2011; 96: F254-7.

Schmiilzer GM, Kamlin CO, Dawson JA, te Pas AB, Morley CJ, Davis PG. Respiratory monitoring of neonatal resuscitation. Arch Dis Child Fetal Neonatal Ed 201 O; 95: F295-303.

Schmolzer GM, Morley CJ, Wong C, Dawson JA, Kamlin CO, Donath SM, et al. Respiratory function monitor guidance of mask ventilation in the delivery room: a feasibility study. J Pediatr 2012;160(3):377-381 e2.

Schmolzer GM, Agarwal M, Kamlin CO, Davis PG. Supraglottic airway devices during neonatal resuscitation: an historical perspective, systematic review and metaanalysis of available clinical trials. Resuscitation 2013; 84: 722-30.

Singh R. Controlled trial to evaluate the use of LMA for neonatal resuscitation. J Anaesth Clin Pharmacol 2005; 21: 303-6.

Tracy MB, Klimek J, Coughtrey H et al. Mask leak in one-person mask ventilation compared to two-person in newborn infant manikin study. Arch Dis Child Fetal Neonatal Ed 2011; 96: F195-200.

Trevisanuto D, Micaglio M, Pillon M, Magarotto M, Piva D, Zanardo V. Laryngeal mask airway: is the management of neonates requiring positive pressure ventilation at birth changing? Resuscitation 2004; 62: 151-7.

Walker R, Ellwood J. The management of the difficult intubation in children. Pediatric Anesthesia 2009; 19(suppl.1): 77-87.

Wilson E, O'Shea J, Thio M, Dawson J, Boland R, Davis P. Arch Dis Child Fetal Neonatal Ed 2014; 99: 2 F169-F171.

Wood FE, Morley CJ, Dawson JA et al. Assessing the effectiveness of two round neonatal resuscitation masks: study 1. Arch Dis Child Fetal Neonatal Ed 2008; 93: F235-7.

Wood FE, Morley CJ, Dawson JA et al. Improved techniques reduce facemask leak during simulated neonatal resuscitation: study 2. Arch Dis Child Fetal Neonatal Ed 2008; 93: F230-4.

Wood FE, Morley CJ, Dawson JA et al. A respiratory function monitor improves mask ventilation. Arch Dis Child Fetal Neonatal Ed 2008; 93: F380-1.

Wyllie J, Perlman J, Kattwinkel J et al. 2010 International consensus on cardiopulmonary resuscitation and emergency cardiovascular care science with treatment recommendations: Neonatal resuscitation. Resuscitation 201 0; 81 S: e260-87.

Zha X, Lin B, Zhang 0, Ye H, Yu R. A prospective evaluation of the efficacy of the laryngeal mask during neonatal resuscitation. Resuscitation 2011; 82: 1405-1409.

Zhu XY, Lin BC, Zhang OS, Ye HM, Yu RJ. A prospective evaluation of the efficacy of the laryngeal mask airway during neonatal resuscitation. Resuscitation 2011; 82: 1405-9.

Singletary EM, Zideman DA, Bendall JC, Berry DA, Borra V, Carlson JN, Cassan P, Chang WT, Charlton NP, Djärv T, Douma MJ, Epstein JL, Hood NA, Markenson DS, Meyran D, Orkin A, Sakamoto T, Swain JM, Woodin JA, De Buck E, De Brier N, O D, Picard C, Goolsby C, Oliver E, Klaassen B, Poole K, Aves T, Lin S, Handley AJ, Jensen J, Allan KS, Lee CC; First Aid Science Collaborators. 2020 International Consensus on First Aid Science With Treatment Recommendations. Resuscitation. 2020 Nov;156:A240-A282. doi.org/10.1016/j.resuscitation.2021.02.014.

O'Shea JE, Scrivens A, Edwards G, Roehr CC. Safe emergency neonatal airway management: current challenges and potential approaches. Arch Dis Child Fetal Neonatal Ed. 2021 Apr 21:fetalneonatal-2020-319398. doi: 10.1136/archdischild-2020-319398. Epub ahead of print. PMID: 33883207.

Calevo MG, Veronese N, Cavallin F, Paola C, Micaglio M, Trevisanuto D. Supraglottic airway devices for surfactant treatment: systematic review and meta-analysis. J Perinatol. 2019 Feb;39(2):173-183. doi: 10.1038/s41372-018-0281-x. Epub 2018 Dec 5. PMID: 30518796.

Cardiovascular problems

In this chapter

Cyanotic and acyanotic congenital heart disease

Persistent pulmonary hypertension of the newborn

Heart failure

Neonatal arrythmias

Inotropes

The learning outcomes will enable you to:

Understand the fetal and postnatal circulation and the role of the arterial duct

Understand the pathophysiology, identification and immediate management of duct-dependent structural congenital heart disease

Have strategies to differentiate cardiac from non-cardiac causes of compromise and collapse

Understand the pathophysiology, identification and immediate management of persistent pulmonary hypertension of the newborn (PPHN)

Understand the pathophysiology of reduced cardiac output and systemic hypotension in a variety of clinical scenarios and have a strategy for appropriate management

Introduction

Congenital heart disease has a reported incidence of around 6–8 per 1000 live births in the UK although more serious abnormalities occur in 2–4 per 1000 depending on definition. The structural lesions which may cause compromise in the newborn infant represent a proportion of these. Additionally, rhythm abnormalities, cardiomyopathies and secondary cardiac compromise may present in the newborn period.

Background

The transition from the fetal to postnatal circulation is one of the key physiological adaptations to occur after birth.

In the fetus, the source of oxygenation is the placenta with only 15% of cardiac output passing through the fetal lungs. This is achieved by means of three separate shunts: the ductus venosus, foramen ovalis and ductus arteriosus.

Oxygenated blood from the placenta passes via the ductus venosus towards the right atrium where it is directed preferentially across the patent foramen ovalis to the left atrium and hence to the left ventricle, aorta and the head and neck vessels. This enables streaming of the most oxygenated blood to the brain and coronary circulation.

Deoxygenated blood returns to the right atrium via the superior vena cava (SVC) and inferior vena cava (IVC). This passes to the right ventricle and on to the main pulmonary artery and then through the widely open ductus arteriosus to join the descending aorta. This right to left shunting through the ductus arteriosus is favoured due to the high pulmonary vascular resistance (PVR) (Figure 8.1).

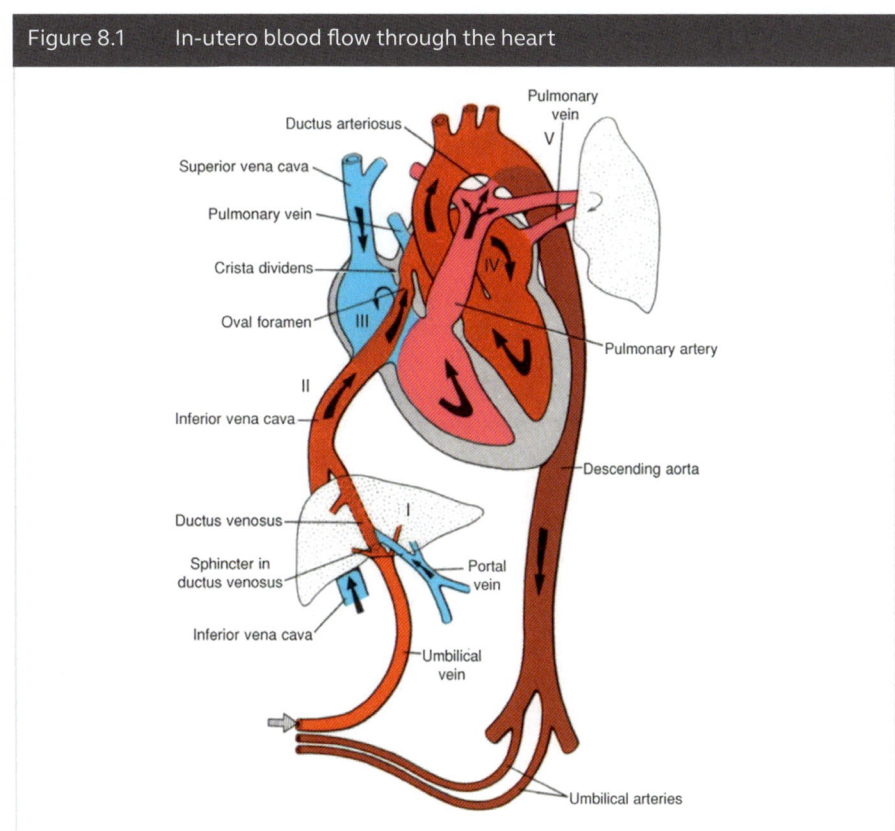

Figure 8.1 In-utero blood flow through the heart

After birth, the placental circulation stops and the lungs are the site of oxygenation. Cessation of blood flow in the umbilical vein results in closure of the ductus venosus and a reduced pressure in the right atrium. In response to expansion of the lungs and increased alveolar oxygen tension, there is a reduction in pulmonary vascular resistance. This gives rise to increased pulmonary blood flow and thus increased return to the left atrium. Now there is increased pressure in the left atrium relative to the right. This pressure difference causes functional closure of the foramen ovalis.

In term babies the ductus arteriosus functionally closes at around 10–15 h post birth. This is primarily in response to increased oxygen tension which stimulates the ductal smooth muscle to constrict. The sensitivity of the ductal smooth muscle to oxygen increases throughout gestation and is less responsive in premature infants.

The ductus arteriosus constricts in response to a decrease in Prostaglandin E2 (PGE2) levels after birth, the placenta being a source of its production and the lungs with more perfusion are now the site of deactivation. Premature infants have higher levels of circulating PGE2. Anatomical closure of the ductus arteriosus in the term infant is usually completed by 14–21 days of postnatal life.

In the newborn infant it is important to understand:
- Pulmonary vascular resistance (PVR) will increase in response to hypoxia and acidosis.
- PVR will decrease in response to effective aeration of the lungs and increased oxygen tension.
- The ductus arteriosus will constrict in response to increased oxygen tension and decreased circulating PGE2.
- The constricting ductus arteriosus will relax in response to hypoxia, acidosis and increased PGE2.
- The premature infant has increased circulating levels of PGE2 and its ductus arteriosus is less responsive to the constricting stimulus of oxygen.

All women in the UK are offered an ultrasound scan at around 20 weeks gestation. The scan is part of the NHS Fetal Anomaly Screening Programme. Basic four chamber cardiac views are obtained. Any suspected anomaly on these views or other high-risk indicators (maternal diabetes, maternal systemic lupus erythromatosis (SLE), family history of congenital heart disease, increased nuchal measurement, various chromosomal abnormalities and syndromes) will result in referral for a fetal cardiac assessment. Whilst the skill and experience of the practitioners performing these fetal echocardiograms has revolutionised prenatal cardiac diagnosis, the transition from fetal to postnatal circulation may unmask previously unidentified abnormalities.

The normal transition from fetal to postnatal circulation will result in a marked clinical deterioration in babies whose circulation is duct dependent. Oxygenation in cases of transposition of the great arteries (TGA) may deteriorate upon ductal closure. Closure of the ductus venous may also cause marked deterioration in certain instances of anomalous pulmonary venous drainage.

The cyanotic baby: distinguishing cyanotic congenital heart disease from respiratory disease in the compromised and sick infant

Respiratory disease, sepsis and neurological compromise predominate as causes of morbidity and mortality on neonatal units. However, it is important to appreciate that cyanotic congenital heart disease (CHD) can present similarly to respiratory illness and sepsis and their differentiation can be problematic.

The importance of this in the context of acute resuscitation of a compromised baby lies not in arriving at the exact diagnosis, but in considering congenital heart disease, instituting appropriate and timely management to prevent further deterioration and referring for expert help.

Table 8.1 Factors that help discriminate between respiratory and cardiac pathology

Factor	Respiratory pathology	Cardiac pathology
History	Prematurity, meconium, difficult delivery	Other congenital abnormalities on antenatal scanning or suspicious fetal heart ultrasound findings
Family history of congenital heart disease		Present
General examination		Relative lack of respiratory distress. Lack of respiratory signs on auscultation
Cardiac examination		+/- heart murmur, parasternal heave, abnormal peripheral pulses
Chest X-ray	Evidence of lung pathology: RDS, pneumothorax, meconium aspiration, infection, congenital diaphragmatic hernia	Decreased or increased pulmonary vascular markings, +/- cardiomegaly, abnormal cardiac silhouette
ECG		Abnormal
Response to 100% oxygen (hyperoxia test)	Significantly increased PaO_2 compared with baseline	Little or no increase in PaO_2 compared with baseline
$PaCO_2$	High	Low or normal

Management will be considered below. Helpful discriminatory clues are shown in Table 8.1. A number of centres in the UK offer pulse oximetry screening to all newborn babies to help identify cases of undiagnosed cyanotic congenital heart disease.

The hyperoxia test

Also known as the nitrogen washout test; it is not absolute however it may be useful if considered in the context of the clinical situation. Increased oxygen delivery will usually increase oxygen saturations if there is a respiratory problem but not if there is a cyanotic congenital cardiac abnormality.

- Measure a pre-test arterial PaO_2.
- Give 100% oxygen for 10 min (caution in premature infants).
- Repeat PaO_2 measurement.
- In cyanosis secondary to respiratory disease, there should be a significant increase in the PaO_2 to levels > 100 mmHg / 14 kPa.
- This test is not absolute and will not be applicable in certain situations (e.g. severe respiratory disease with large intrapulmonary shunting, anomalous venous drainage and others).

Duct dependent congenital heart disease – physiology, recognition and management

Closure of the ductus arteriosus is a normal physiological adaptation to postnatal life which takes place functionally in the term newborn infant at 10–15 h after birth. In those infants with duct dependent congenital heart disease, the closure of the ductus arteriosus may herald a marked deterioration and collapse. The diagnosis of congenital heart disease should be considered promptly as appropriate management must be initiated without delay.

It can be difficult to differentiate this situation from others such as sepsis in the collapsed infant and PPHN in the cyanosed infant.

The duct dependent circulation can be categorised into three types:

1. Duct dependent systemic circulation
2. Duct dependent pulmonary circulation
3. Duct dependent mixing.

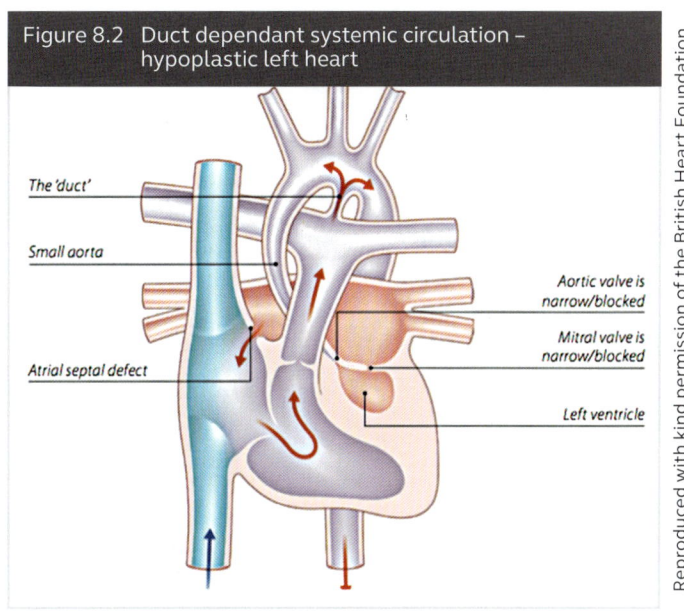

Figure 8.2 Duct dependant systemic circulation – hypoplastic left heart

1. Duct dependent systemic circulation

In this situation forward flow in the descending aorta is dependent on right to left shunting through the arterial duct. This occurs when forward flow from the left ventricle through the left ventricular outflow tract or through the ascending aorta and arch is obstructed. Conditions include critical aortic stenosis, interrupted aortic arch, hypoplastic left heart syndrome (Figure 8.2) and coarctation of the aorta.

Constriction and closure of the ductus arteriosus after birth compromises the systemic circulation. This presents with worsening perfusion, progressive metabolic acidosis and systemic hypotension and collapse, usually within a few days of birth.

Helpful indicators may include:

- weak or absent femoral pulses
- blood pressure in right arm > blood pressure in the legs
- pre-ductal saturation, (measured on the right arm) ≥ 5% higher than post ductal saturation, (measured on the legs)*
- a difference of greater than 10–15 mmHg/1.5–2 kPa between PaO_2 measured pre-ductally, (right radial artery) and post ductally (UAC)*
- murmur on cardiac examination
- abnormal ECG
- absence of signs of sepsis, metabolic disease or other respiratory pathology.

*This can be observed in both PPHN (see below) and some left ventricular outflow tract obstructive lesions (e.g. interrupted aortic arch, coarctation).

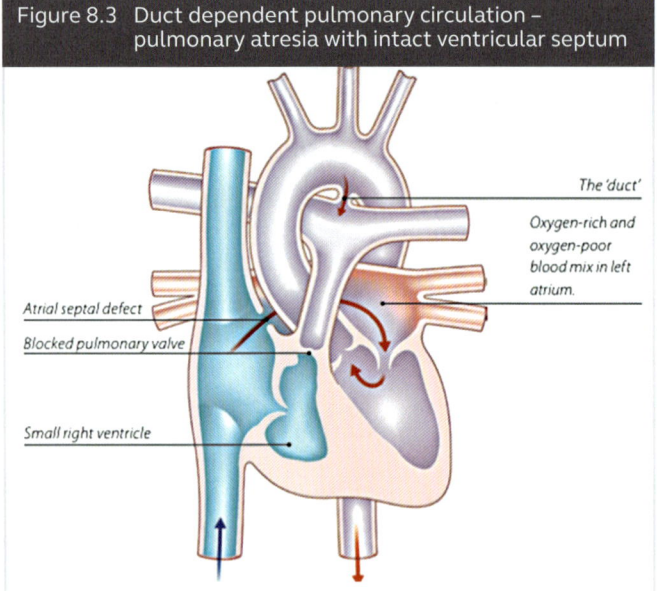

Figure 8.3 Duct dependent pulmonary circulation – pulmonary atresia with intact ventricular septum

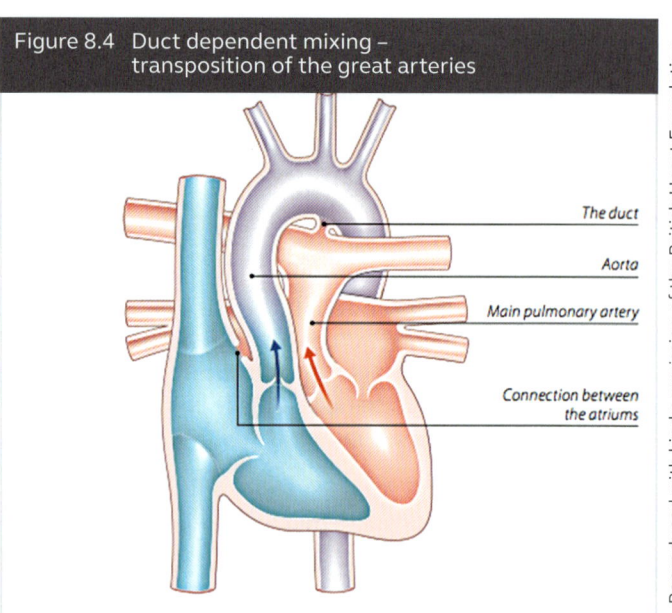

Figure 8.4 Duct dependent mixing – transposition of the great arteries

2. Duct dependent pulmonary circulation

In this situation forward flow to the lungs is dependent on left to right shunting through the ductus arteriosus. This occurs when forward flow from the right side of the heart through the right ventricular outflow tract to the pulmonary arteries is compromised or obstructed.

Lesions leading to a duct dependent pulmonary circulation include tricuspid atresia with intact ventricular septum, pulmonary atresia (Figure 8.3) and critical pulmonary stenosis.

Constriction and closure of the ductus arteriosus compromises the pulmonary circulation and causes progressive cyanosis, often in the absence of respiratory signs, leading to acidosis and collapse.

Indicators include:

- Normal or low $PaCO_2$ in the presence of hypoxaemia
- Relative failure to respond by significantly increasing PaO_2 following administration of high inspired oxygen concentrations for 10 min or longer (hyperoxia test)
- Chest X-ray abnormalities especially pulmonary oligaemia
- ECG abnormalities
- Murmur on cardiac examination
- Relative lack of respiratory distress given degree of hypoxaemia.

3. Duct dependent mixing

Certain conditions such as transposition of the great arteries (TGA) (Figure 8.4) may be dependent on the ductus arteriosus for mixing of the pulmonary and systemic circulations. Without mixing these would otherwise exist as two independent circuits. TGA is often associated with the presence of ventricular septal defects and there is a communication between the two atria at birth. If these communications are small however, constriction of the duct will lead to progressive cyanosis and compromise. Ductal patency must be maintained until expert cardiological management, usually in the form of an atrial septostomy, can be instituted.

Management of the duct-dependent circulation

Use the ARNI algorithm: ABC assessment, then an ABCDEF approach to institute resuscitation.

- Consider the diagnosis of congenital heart disease.
- Start intravenous prostaglandin infusion.
- Obtain expert advice from a paediatric cardiologist.

Prostaglandin therapy

Indication – to maintain patency of the ductus arteriosus.

Preparations

- Prostaglandin E1 (Alprostadil) dose = 5 nanograms kg^{-1} min^{-1} and adjust according to response in increments of 5 nanograms kg^{-1} min^{-1} to maximum 100 nanograms kg^{-1} min^{-1} (side effects increase with higher doses).
- Prostaglandin E2 (Dinoprostone) dose = 5 nanograms kg^{-1} min^{-1}.
Increase in increments of 5 nanograms kg^{-1} min^{-1} to a maximum of 20 nanograms kg^{-1} min^{-1} again anticipating increasing side effects.

Side effects of prostaglandin

- Apnoea
- Bradycardia
- Hypotension
- Pyrexia
- Flushing
- Jitteriness
- Convulsions
- Diarrhoea.

Side effects particularly with increasing doses must be anticipated. Intubation and ventilation may be required for prolonged or persistent apnoeas. This may be particularly relevant if the baby is about to be transported in an ambulance to a cardiac centre. Continuous monitoring of heart rate, respiratory rate, blood pressure and temperature are required. Stopping the infusion and restarting at a lower dose will usually relieve side effects. Do not flush a line containing a prostaglandin preparation.

Persistent pulmonary hypertension of the newborn infant

In this condition there is persistence of high pulmonary vascular resistance after birth leading to cyanosis from right to left shunting at ductal and atrial levels.

The heart is structurally normal.

Causes of pulmonary hypertension

- Pulmonary vasoconstriction secondary to factors such as hypoxia, hypothermia, acidosis and pain
- Decreased size of pulmonary vascular bed
- Chronic hypertrophy of pulmonary vascular smooth muscle in utero.

PPHN can be caused by a number of conditions. Meconium aspiration syndrome is a common cause. Sepsis, especially Group B Streptococcal sepsis and birth asphyxia can lead to hypoxia and PPHN. Respiratory distress syndrome, pulmonary hypoplasia and congenital diaphragmatic hernia are often associated with pulmonary hypertension.

Clinical presentation

- Respiratory distress.
- Difficulty in achieving oxygenation – may be out of proportion to relative ease of maintaining normal $PaCO_2$.
- Significantly higher pre-ductal saturations or PaO_2 (measured from the right arm) compared with post ductal saturations or PaO_2.*
- Chest X-ray may demonstrate the primary respiratory pathology.

* NB this does not differentiate PPHN from congenital heart disease with right to left shunting.

Goals of management

These management principles are specific to optimising the condition of the baby in the acute setting of PPHN and assume emergency and general supportive management is already in place.

The goals of management of the baby with PPHN involve strategies for reducing pulmonary vascular resistance based on the physiological principles discussed above:

- Optimise oxygenation – high inhaled oxygen concentration, optimising ventilation. High frequency oscillation ventilation may be effective. Sedation and muscle relaxation.
- Avoid and correct acidosis – aim for a pH in the normal range. Do not aim for alkalosis or hypocapnia as this causes cerebral vasoconstriction.
- Use inotropes to maintain a blood pressure (BP) with a mean value 5–10 higher than the mean for gestational age to discourage right to left shunting across the ductus arteriosus. An echocardiogram can be helpful to guide BP parameters and inotrope selection.
- Maintain a normal glucose, calcium and magnesium.
- Correct polycythaemia.
- Consider inhaled nitric oxide therapy as a potent and selective pulmonary vasodilator (10–20 ppm).

Heart failure in the newborn infant

Heart failure may occur due to a variety of causes, both congenital and acquired. Those presenting in the neonatal period will be considered.

Common causes of neonatal heart failure

- Structural heart disease causing volume overload – the time of onset of congestive heart failure can be predicted from the type of abnormality. It would be unusual for large left to right shunts from PDA or VSD to give rise to heart failure at less than 6 weeks of age except in preterm babies. Lesions presenting within the first week would include hypoplastic left heart syndrome, severe tricuspid or pulmonary regurgitation, large systemic arteriovenous malformations, TGA and anomalous pulmonary venous drainage especially if obstructed.
- Disease of the cardiac muscle – cardiomyopathies.
- Damage to the heart muscle, (e.g. hypoxia in HIE).
- Biochemical problems: hypoxia, acidosis, hypoglycaemia and hypocalcaemia.
- Arrhythmias – Supraventricular tachycardia or complete heart block.
- Severe anaemia.

Heart failure presentation

- Respiratory distress, poor feeding, clamminess, sweating, especially on feeding.
- Excessive weight gain (normal = 30 g per day in a term baby).
- Tachypnoea, respiratory distress, tachycardia, gallop rhythm and hepatomegaly. Oedema is unusual.
- Chest X-ray changes include cardiomegaly and diffuse increase in opacity of the lung fields, fluid in the horizontal fissure +/- small pulmonary effusions.
- ECG – may show a right sided overload / strain pattern or rhythm abnormalities according to the underlying cause.

Management of heart failure

Initial assessment of ABC with management of immediate problems and subsequent ABCDEF approach to resuscitation should be adopted with appropriate support being requested. Additional management points include:

- Aim for a biochemical environment in which cardiac function is optimised: avoid acidosis, hypoxia and achieve normal levels of glucose, potassium, calcium and magnesium.
- Identify and treat arrhythmias.
- Achieve good oxygenation but avoid hyperoxia which will lower pulmonary vascular resistance increasing any left to right shunting.
- Diuretics – furosemide 1–2 mg kg^{-1} IV.
- Consider inotrope infusion (Table 8.2).
- Careful assessment of the need for fluid boluses, avoiding fluid overload.
- Consider if prostaglandin is indicated.
- Paediatric cardiology opinion for ongoing investigations and management.

Neonatal arrhythmias

Supra ventricular tachycardia is the commonest neonatal arrhythmia. Atrial flutter and complete heart block occur less frequently but may require emergency management in the newborn period.

Neonatal arrhythmias may be diagnosed prenatally and if they occur for a significant duration in fetal life they may lead to antenatal heart failure and hydrops fetalis.

Supraventricular tachycardia (SVT)

This is the commonest arrhythmia in infancy and typically gives rise to a narrow complex tachycardia with a rate usually greater than 220 bpm. It must be differentiated from sinus tachycardia. Helpful differentiating features include the following:

- In sinus tachycardia the heart rate may vary with stimulation of the baby and from beat to beat but this is not the case in SVT.
- Termination of SVT is abrupt however HR gradually slows in sinus tachycardia with treatment.

SVT may originate secondary to an atrial or less commonly a junctional ectopic focus, or due to an AV re-entry circuit.

The presentation of SVT in the newborn infant is variable and it may be very well tolerated. SVT may revert spontaneously or may present with heart failure particularly if the tachycardia is sustained. It is important to establish the diagnosis with an ECG (Figure 8.5). It is imperative to print and record rhythm strips of the arrhythmia during any intervention or treatment which may be given.

Emergency management of SVT

This is indicated in symptomatic infants or in those with heart failure.

- Record pre-treatment ECG.
- Obtain advice, as required, from a paediatric cardiologist.
- Record an ECG rhythm strip during each of the following manoeuvres.

Vagal manoeuvres

The most effective and appropriate vagal manoeuvre in infants is facial immersion in cold water or placing a plastic bag filled with iced water on the face.

Adenosine

Adenosine should be given by a rapid IV bolus. The half-life is less than 10 s and a reliable cannula in a large vein is needed. A starting dose of 150 microgram kg^{-1} is recommended, followed by a generous flush. Further doses may be needed. The dose should be incrementally increased by 50 microgram kg^{-1} until reversion to sinus rhythm occurs or a maximum dose of 250 microgram kg^{-1} is reached. Adenosine interrupts A-V conduction and there is often a brief period of no electrical activity followed by nodal escape and a bradycardia before eventual restoration of sinus rhythm. Side effects include sinus bradycardia, AV block, bronchial constriction, flushing and agitation. Full resuscitation equipment must be available.

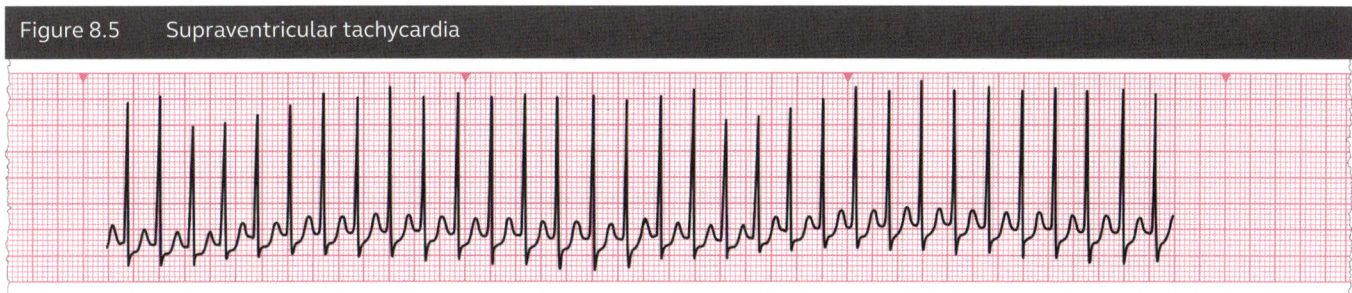

Figure 8.5 Supraventricular tachycardia

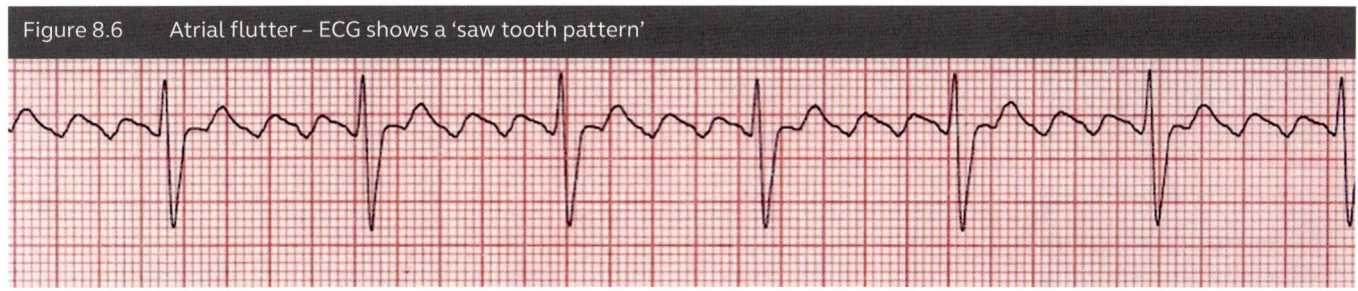

Figure 8.6 Atrial flutter – ECG shows a 'saw tooth pattern'

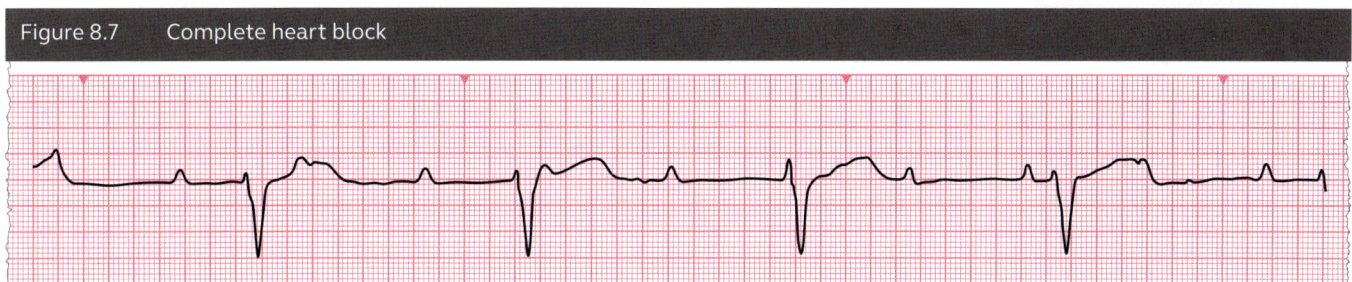

Figure 8.7 Complete heart block

Synchronised cardioversion

Synchronised cardioversion under sedation or general anaesthetic may be required immediately in the severely compromised infant or if drug therapy fails. Start with an energy of 0.5 J kg^{-1} increasing if unsuccessful incrementally to 2 J kg^{-1}.

Atrial flutter

Atrial flutter may arise in fetal life. This can present prenatally or in the newborn period. Heart rates of around 300 bpm may occur, causing heart failure and hydrops fetalis.

Atrial flutter can look similar to an SVT (Figure 8.6). Adenosine will not convert this arrhythmia to sinus rhythm but its action to temporarily block the AV node may be useful in unmasking the underlying flutter.

Emergency management proceeds with the ABC, ABCDEF approach to newborn resuscitation with specific management to include:

- Confirm diagnosis by ECG.
- Record rhythm strips during any intervention.
- Obtain advice from a paediatric cardiologist.
- In the severely compromised infant with heart failure, immediate synchronised DC cardioversion is indicated.

Complete heart block

The incidence of congenital complete heart block is approximately 1 in 20 000 live births. It can be associated with structural heart abnormalities and maternal SLE, particularly in the presence of anti-Ro and anti-La antibodies.

Complete heart block presents variably ranging from asymptomatic to significant heart failure. Those infants presenting in heart failure should have emergency management instituted following the ARNI approach to newborn resuscitation.

Management of complete heart block includes confirmation of the diagnosis by ECG (Figure 8.7), may include the use of diuretics and inotropes as appropriate, and the use of isoprenaline to increase the heart rate. Expert paediatric cardiology advice will be needed.

Further management will include echocardiography to identify structural heart disease and consideration of cardiac pacing. Pacing is generally indicated in symptomatic infants and those with heart rates less than 55 beats per minute.

Figure 8.8 Causes and management of hypotension

Hypovlaemia / APH / Other acute blood loss / Redistribution
→ Management: Re-establishment of normovolaemia 10–20 mL kg^{-1} 0.9% sodium chloride / blood. Repeat as indicated

Depressed myocardial function
→ Management: See management of heart failure and inotrope sections in this chapter

Duct dependant systemic circulation / Left ventricular outflow tract obstruction
→ Management: See management of heart failure and inotrope sections in this chapter

Vasodilation sepsis
→ Management: Consider volume resuscitation and see inotrope guided intrope section (Table 8.2)

Neurological

The hypotensive infant

The common causes of acute hypotension in the neonate are summarised in Figure 8.8. Management is dependent upon the cause and its pathophysiology.

Inotropes

Indications for the use of inotropic agents in newborn resuscitation are discussed in Figure 8.8. The most suitable drug is determined by the pathophysiological state of the baby's heart, circulation and the effects one wishes to achieve (Table 8.2).

The pharmacological effects of these drugs are summarised below followed by a suggestion as to which agent to use when.

- In a clinical state where vasodilation predominates, (e.g. early sepsis), increasing the systemic vascular resistance may be desirable and it might be helpful to consider dopamine in the higher dose range, adrenaline or noradrenaline.

- In low cardiac output states, (e.g. cardiogenic shock) dobutamine, adrenaline or with expert advice, milrinone could be considered.

- In hypovolaemic shock in addition to treating with adequate volume replacement and addressing any ongoing causes, the addition of higher doses of dopamine or use of adrenaline might be helpful.

It is important to recognise the differing pharmacological effects of different inotropic drugs. Their use should be tailored to an individual clinical situation.

Table 8.2 Properties of different inotropes

Inotrope	Dose	Mode of action	Systolic function	Diastolic function	SVR	PVR	Heart rate
Dopamine	1–5 micrograms kg mins^{-1}	Dopamine Receptors	Minimal +	–	–	–	+
Dopamine	6–10 micrograms kg mins^{-1}	B1 agonist	+	–	+	Minimal +	+
Dopamine	11–20 micrograms kg mins^{-1}	alpha agonist	+	–	++	Minimal ++	+
Dobutamine	1–20 micrograms kg mins^{-1}	B1 agonist alpha antagonist	+	–	Decrease	Minimal decrease	+
Adrenaline		B1 agonist > alpha agonist	++	–	+	Minimal +	+
Nor-adrenaline		alpha agonist > B1 agonist	+	–	++	Minimal +	+
Milrinone		Phosphodiesterase inhibitor	+	+	Decrease	Decrease	–

– indicates 'no effect'
SVR = systemic vascular resistance
PVC = pulmonary vascular resistance

08: Summary learning

It is important to consider cardiovascular causes of compromise and collapse in the newborn infant.

It may be difficult to differentiate cardiac from non-cardiac causes of compromise especially sepsis, respiratory disease and PPHN. Helpful indicators are discussed.

Certain structural heart conditions are dependent on the patency of the ductus arteriosus. Prompt recognition and management of congenital heart disease is important.

Heart failure in the newborn infant may be due to a variety of causes and appropriate initial management is described.

The use of inotropes in the neonate should be tailored to the individual situation.

My key take-home messages from this chapter are:

Further reading

Archer N, Burch M. Paediatric Cardiology – An Introduction. Part Two – Cardiac Problems in Infancy. London: Chapman & Hall. 1998.

Boyle E, Cusack J. Emergency topics and controversies in Neonatology. London Springer 2020, chapters 6-7.

British Heart Foundation. 'Understanding Your Child's Heart'. www.bhf.org.uk/publications.aspx

Park MK. Pediatric Cardiology for Practitioners, 5th Edition. Chapter 8 Fetal and Perinatal Circulation. Philadelphia, Mosby Elsevier: 2008.

Neonatal surgical conditions

09

In this chapter

Congenital and acquired neonatal surgical conditions

Neonatal surgical emergencies

Consideration of associated anomalies

The learning outcomes will enable you to:

Assess and initiate the management of babies with commonly encountered surgical conditions

Predict likely problems and worrying features

Identify neonatal surgical emergencies

Introduction

With improved antenatal screening a large proportion, but not all, congenital surgical anomalies are now diagnosed antenatally. If so, a plan can be put in place, regarding timing and place of delivery. However, this will not always be the case. Hence, ARNI providers need to be able to provide the initial stabilisation.

Intestinal obstruction (e.g. oesophageal atresia, duodenal atresia, ileal atresia) may present with polyhydramnios antenatally. Many congenital defects are obvious at delivery. This chapter deals with common neonatal surgical conditions and surgical emergencies (e.g. volvulus) that require special measures at delivery or prompt management in the newborn period.

Tracheoesophageal fistula and oesophageal atresia

Incidence	1 in 3500 births. Various types as shown in Figure 9.1.
Antenatal features	May have polyhydramnios and absent stomach bubble.
Postnatal presentation	Increased secretions, choking with feeds and difficulty passing a nasogastric tube.
Assessment and initial actions	Secretions may cause airway compromise or aspiration pneumonia.
	Continuous suction of the oesophageal pouch may be needed; a replogle tube is designed to do this.
	CPAP may cause progressive abdominal distension and should be avoided if possible as you cannot aspirate air from the stomach.
	Chest and abdominal X-ray with a nasogastric tube (NGT) in place, will show the coiled NGT in the oesophageal pouch, confirming the diagnosis of oesophageal atresia. The presence of air in the stomach indicates a distal tracheo-esophageal fistula.
	Assess for associated features e.g. VACTERL association which includes Vertebral anomalies (e.g. hemivertebrae), Anorectal malformation, Cardiac anomalies, TE (Tracheo-Esophageal atresia), Renal and Limb abnormalities.
	Chest and abdominal X-ray with a nasogastric tube (NGT) in place, will show the coiled NGT in the oesophageal pouch, confirming the diagnosis of oesophageal atresia. The presence of air in the stomach indicates a distal tracheo-esophageal fistula.
Important features	Check for signs of airway compromise due to secretions or bronchomalacia.
	Check for signs of aspiration.
	Assess for signs of associated congenital heart disease.
	Abdominal distension can cause respiratory compromise.

Figure 9.1 Incidence of different types of tracheoesophageal fistula and oesophageal atresia

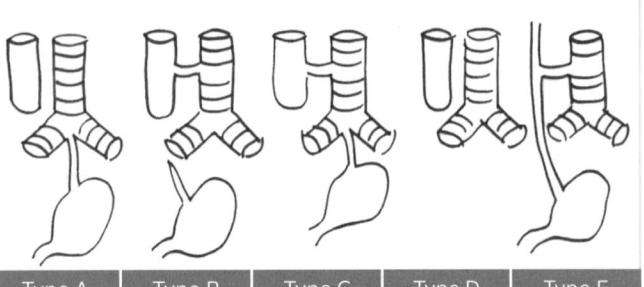

Type A	Oesophageal atresia with distal fistula	incidence 85%
Type B	Oesophageal atresia with proximal fistula	incidence 2%
Type C	Oesophageal atresia with proximal and distal fistula	incidence < 1%
Type D	Oesophageal atresia with no tracheoesophageal fistula	incidence 8%
Type E	H-type tracheoesophageal fistula	incidence 4%

Duodenal atresia

Incidence	1 in 8000 births.
Antenatal features	Polyhydramnios and double bubble on fetal ultrasound.
Postnatal presentation	Vomiting or increased nasogastric aspirates which may be bile stained.
Assessment and initial actions	Airway secretions may cause compromise.
	Pass a wide bore nasogastric tube placed on free drainage, and regularly aspirate stomach contents.
	Assess fluid status if vomiting has been significant.
	Assess for associated features. Duodenal atresia is one of several intestinal birth defects that occur more frequently in infants with Trisomy 21 and associated problems, (e.g. congenital heart disease), need to be sought and excluded.
	X-rays show a characteristic 'double bubble' appearance (Figure 9.2)
Important features	Check for signs of airway compromise or signs of aspiration.
	Signs of cyanotic congenital heart disease.
	Assess for signs of hypovolaemia and dehydration if vomiting has been severe.

Figure 9.2 X-ray of duodenal atresia showing a 'double bubble'

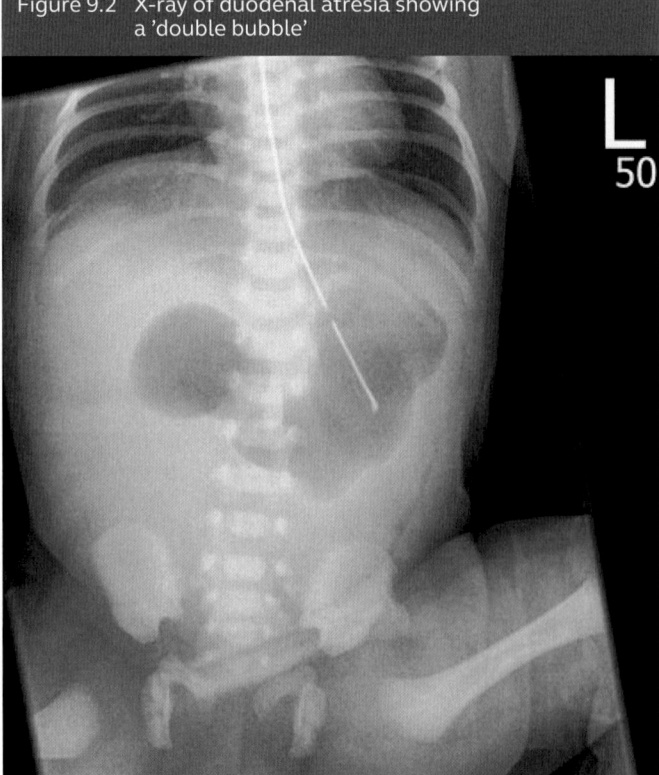

Ischaemic bowel and volvulus

Incidence	Rare.
Antenatal features	Often not diagnosed antenatally – may have dilated loops of bowel.
Postnatal presentation	Abdominal distension +/- tenderness, bilious vomiting, shock.
Assessment and initial actions	Acute volvulus can present with shock and significant cardiorespiratory compromise. The initial assessment may show potentially life-threatening features. Consider intubation and ventilation. Babies with volvulus are likely to need fluid resuscitation. This is a **surgical emergency** and urgent surgical intervention is needed following rapid stabilisation as this can prevent significant bowel loss. Arrange transfer to an appropriate unit if required.
Important features	Check for signs of acute cardiovascular compromise. Babies with an acute surgical abdomen are likely to need significant resuscitation and may need volume support and inotropes prior to theatre.

Abdominal wall defects: gastroschisis and exomphalos

Incidence	1 in 2000 births.
Antenatal features	Abdominal wall defects are usually seen on antenatal scans.
Postnatal presentation	Bowel is seen outside of the abdominal cavity it may be exposed (gastroschisis) or enclosed in a sac (exomphalos).
Assessment and initial actions	**Gastroschisis** Check the colour of the bowel: the mesentery can twist causing ischaemia. Supporting the bowel on the side (Figure 9.3a) can help prevent this until a silo is put in place Fluid can be lost rapidly through the bowel by evaporation. Place the baby in a plastic bag or cover the bowel with 'cling film' to prevent this. Fluid replacement will be necessary. Early surgical correction, either as a primary repair or by placing the bowel in a silo (Figure 9.3b) is indicated. **Exomphalos** Assess for associated genetic conditions: exomphalos is associated with chromosomal disorders. Fluid replacement of NG losses will be necessary. If the sac ruptures, manage as per gastroschisis.
Important features	Check for signs of bowel compromise and ischaemia. Metabolic acidosis suggests inadequate fluid replacement. Assess for signs of associated congenital heart disease (common with exomphalos). Monitor for signs of abdominal compartment syndrome following surgical repair of gastroschisis. This is a rare but important complication which is a **surgical emergency** needing the abdomen to be re-opened.

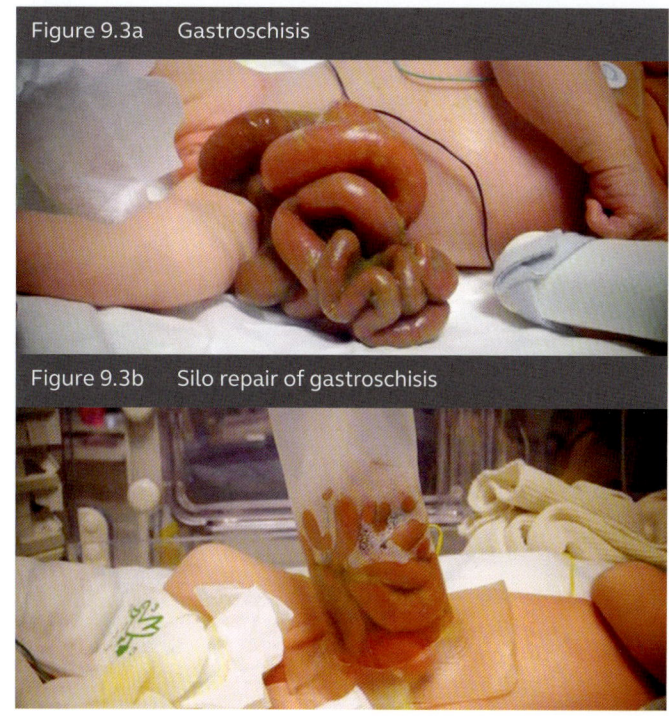

Figure 9.3a Gastroschisis

Figure 9.3b Silo repair of gastroschisis

Congenital diaphragmatic hernia (CDH)

Incidence	1 in 2000 to 1 in 5000 births.
Antenatal features	Approximately 50% cases of congenital diaphragmatic hernia are now diagnosed antenatally. A number of antenatal features can be used to help predict prognosis.
Postnatal presentation	CDH is more common on the left side (Figure 9.4). If not diagnosed antenatally CDH will present with early respiratory distress, unequal air entry and a scaphoid appearance to the abdomen.
Assessment and initial actions	Stabilisation of a baby with CDH is challenging; you will need senior help. Avoid mask ventilation, if possible, as this may cause distension of the bowel in the chest. Early intubation is required. A nasogastric tube should be passed to decompress the bowel. Sedation and muscle relaxants are often used – some units routinely give muscle relaxants on delivery suite. Babies with CDH often develop pulmonary hypertension. Gentle ventilation strategies should be used where possible. Treatment is surgical, once the baby has been stable for a period of time.
Important features	Babies with CDH will need significant intensive care and stabilisation in a tertiary centre. The postnatal mortality is approximately 35%.

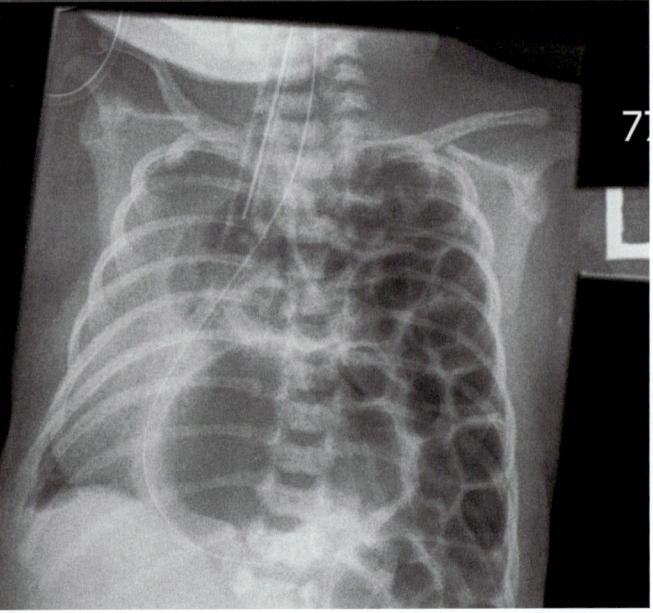

Figure 9.4 X-ray showing congenital left sided diaphragmatic hernia

Spina bifida/myelomeningocoele

Incidence	1 in 6500 births.
Antenatal features	Often diagnosed antenatally: may be associated with hydrocephalus.
Postnatal presentation	Typical spinal lesion seen (see Figure 9.5).
Assessment and initial actions	Most babies do not need resuscitation. Dry and wrap the baby, but be careful not to disturb the sac. Placing the baby on its side will reduce the pressure on the spinal cord. If the lesion is open cover with 0.9% sodium chloride soaked gauze and liaise with a neurosurgical team.
Important features	Check for associated congenital anomalies. Hydrocephalus is a frequent association with spina bifida; the large head may cause delivery problems if it occurs antenatally, postnatally it may impact on airway management and resuscitation decisions. Babies with spina bifida often have bowel and bladder problems, although these are not usually a problem in the first few days. Multidisciplinary input will be needed.

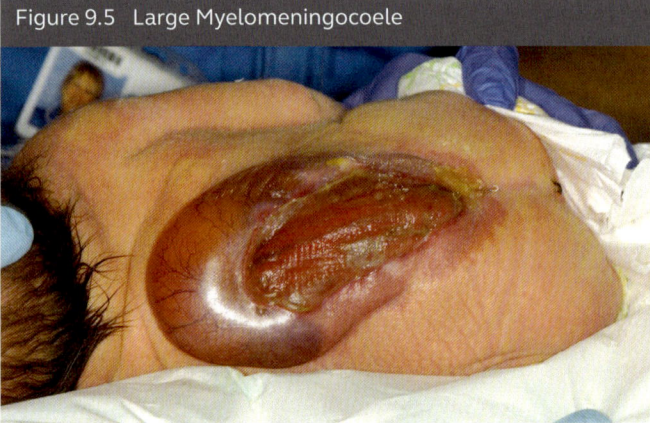

Figure 9.5 Large Myelomeningocoele

Necrotising enterocolitis

Necrotising enterocolitis (NEC) is a common serious complication of prematurity. The aetiology is unknown but there are a number of risk factors:
- prematurity
- abnormal antenatal umbilical artery doppler flow
- intra-uterine growth restriction
- patent ductus arteriosus
- not receiving breast milk
- rapid increase in enteral feeds
- blood transfusions – especially exchange transfusion.

NEC is inversely related to gestational age. It is commoner in smaller and more preterm babies. Less commonly, it can occur in term babies particularly those with intrauterine growth restriction or peripartum compromise. It usually occurs after enteral feeding has been introduced.

Clinical features

NEC may have a rapid or an insidious onset. Any preterm baby with a clinical deterioration should be assessed promptly and the abdomen should be examined. Symptoms include:
- increase in the number of apnoeas and bradycardias
- tachycardia with poor perfusion
- temperature instability
- feed intolerance – an increase in the volume of nasogastric aspirates
- nasogastric aspirates containing bile
- abdominal distension, redness or tenderness
- blood or mucus in the stool
- shock.

Clinical examination may show:
- distended tender abdomen
- redness of the abdominal wall
- a palpable abdominal mass
- cardiovascular compromise.

Severity of NEC can be staged using modified Bell's criteria or other scoring systems. However, these are mainly used in research settings. It is best to describe the clinical features of the baby's condition and the X-ray (Figures 9.6 and 9.7).

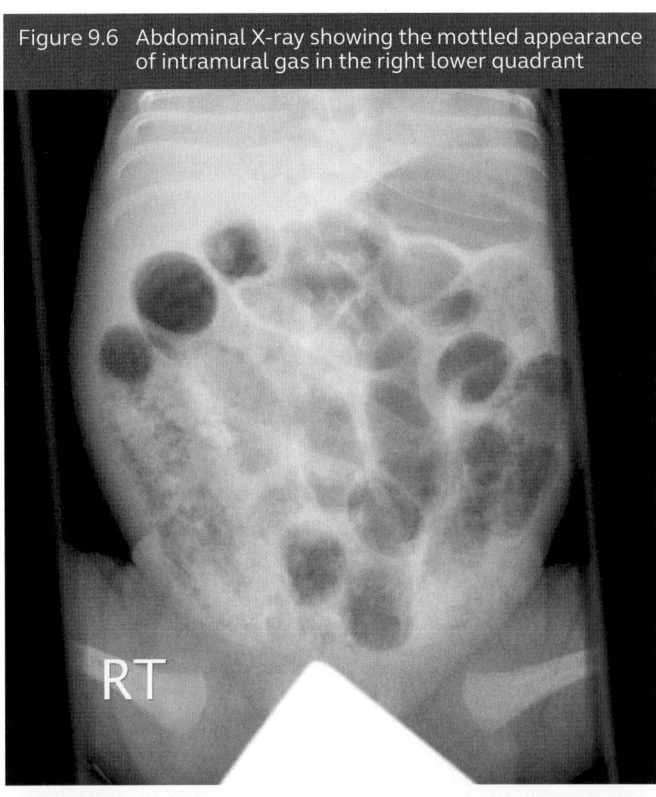

Figure 9.6 Abdominal X-ray showing the mottled appearance of intramural gas in the right lower quadrant

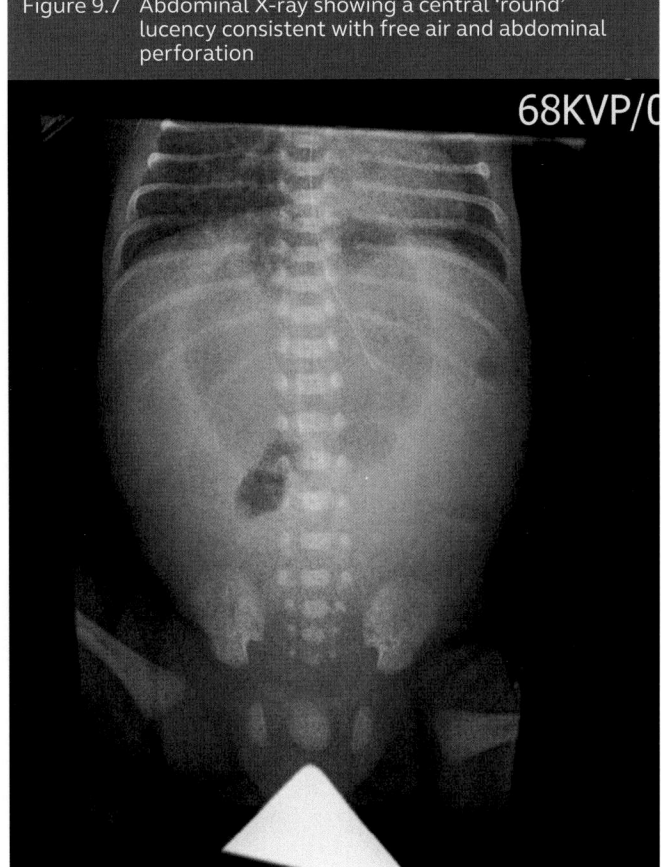

Figure 9.7 Abdominal X-ray showing a central 'round' lucency consistent with free air and abdominal perforation

Initial stabilisation

A Airway and breathing may be compromised by significant abdominal distension. Blood gases should be measured.

B Babies with significant NEC may deteriorate quickly, consider elective intubation and ventilation if the clinical picture is rapidly evolving.

C Babies with NEC often develop hypovolaemic shock. Assess heart rate, capillary refill and blood pressure. An arterial line should be sited if there is concern about cardiovascular status. Babies with acute NEC often need significant volume resuscitation and inotropic support. A central venous line should be inserted for intravenous nutrition and inotropes.

D Babies with NEC often deteriorate quickly, analgesia should be provided and a sick baby may need sedation and muscle relaxation in order to achieve stabilisation. Antibiotics should be administered following local prescribing guidance and should include anaerobic cover.

E Once stable, an abdominal X-ray should be performed to look for radiological signs of NEC (see Figures 9.6 and 9.7).

F A baby with NEC can deteriorate rapidly, be extremely unstable and sometimes requires surgery. This will be a very worrying and distressing time for the parents.

Abdominal X-ray findings include:

- signs of bowel obstruction
- abnormal gas patterns including intramural gas (see Figure 9.6)
- gas in the portal circulation
- signs of perforation (i.e. free gas (see Figure 9.7)).

Blood investigations should be sent for:

- full blood count – there may be anaemia, high or low white cell count or low platelets
- coagulation studies – babies with NEC often have deranged clotting and may need treatment with blood products
- blood cultures
- cross match
- U&E's - fluid resuscitation may lead to electrolyte disturbances, and if an operation is needed, recent electrolytes will help the anaesthetist
- inflammatory markers e.g. CRP as trends over future readings many help indicate disease activity.

Definitive management

The majority of cases of NEC are managed medically. However, if this is unable to maintain bowel viability then surgical resection of disease bowel may be necessary.

Babies should not be fed and intravenous nutrition will be needed. Broad spectrum antibiotics should be administered including anaerobic cover. Babies should be monitored closely to ensure that their clinical and haematological status improves.

Surgical management

The timing of surgical intervention can be difficult and close liaison with surgical colleagues is needed. Laparotomy should be considered if there is a failure to respond to medical treatment or signs of perforation. Emergency surgery can be life-saving in babies that are difficult to stabilise in the initial period. In babies that are too unstable to go to theatre, insertion of a peritoneal drain on the neonatal unit, usually by a surgeon, can help stabilise the baby enough to get them to theatre.

General post-operative care

Babies returning to the neonatal unit from surgery should have a full ABCDEF assessment when they return from theatre. Important considerations are a review of cardiorespiratory support, fluid balance including urine output, analgesia and abdominal compartment syndrome after abdominal surgery. Review any specific postoperative instruction shared by the surgical team.

09: Summary learning

Many, but not all, surgical conditions are now diagnosed in the antenatal period.

The principles of stabilisation follow the standard ARNI algorithm.

Managing the fluid balance and giving appropriate analgesia are important.

Volvulus is a neonatal surgical emergency, requiring rapid stabilisation and urgent discussion with surgical colleagues.

Following stabilisation, liaise with paediatric surgical colleagues and arrange transfer to an appropriate centre for definitive care.

My key take-home messages from this chapter are:

Further reading

British Association of Perinatal Medicine (2018) National Care Principles for the Management of Congenital Diagphragmatic Hernia A BAPM Framework for Practice. https://www.bapm.org/resources/22-national-care-principles-for-the-management-of-congenital-diagphragmatic-hernia-2018

Long A, Bunch KJ, Knight M On behalf of BAPS-CASS, et al Early population-based outcomes of infants born with congenital diaphragmatic hernia Archives of Disease in Childhood - Fetal and Neonatal Edition 2018;103:F517-F522.

Snoek KG, Reiss IK, Greenough A, et al. Standardized Postnatal Management of Infants with Congenital Diaphragmatic Hernia in Europe: The CDH EURO Consortium Consensus - 2015 Update. Neonatology 2016;110(1):66-74.

Gordon PV, Swanson JR, Attridge JT, Clark R. Emerging trends in acquired neonatal intestinal disease: is it time to abandon Bell's criteria? J Perinatol 2007; 27: 667-671.

Logan JW, Rice HE, Goldberg RN, Cotten CM. Congenital diaphragmatic hernia: a systematic review and summary of best-evidence practice strategies. J Perinatol 2007; 27: 535-549.

Shaw-Smith C. Oesophageal atresia, tracheo-oesophageal fistula, and the VACTERL association: review of genetics and epidemiology. J Med Genet 2006; 43: 545-54.

Sepsis

In this chapter

Common organisms causing neonatal sepsis

Risk factors and clinical indicators of early and late onset neonatal sepsis

Investigation and treatment considerations in neonatal sepsis

The learning outcomes will enable you to:

Be aware of the common organisms that cause neonatal sepsis

Be able to identify infants at risk of sepsis

Be able to describe the clinical indicators of neonatal infection

Be able to recognise the 'red flag' signs of serious neonatal infection

Be able to use the ARNI algorithm to stabilise an infant presenting with signs of serious infection

Understand the importance of early antibiotic administration

Introduction

Sepsis is a leading cause of neonatal morbidity and mortality.

Most babies treated on a neonatal unit will receive antibiotics and often preterm babies receive multiple courses of antibiotics during their stay. Newborn babies are exposed to a unique set of organisms from the birth canal, often different from organisms affecting older children and adults. Preterm babies have an immature immune system making them more susceptible to infection and less able to mount an effective immune response.

The overall incidence of serious neonatal infection is around 8 per 1000 live births. Preterm babies are particularly at risk and the incidence rises in a preterm population to between 160 and 300 per 1000 very low birth weight babies.

Neonatal sepsis is traditionally divided into early and late infections. This distinction can be useful as early and late infections can present in different ways and are due to different micro-organisms. There is no single definition of early neonatal infection. Early onset neonatal infection often refers to infection that presents within the first 72 h of life.

Around 30% of women in the UK carry Group B Streptococci (Streptococcus agalactiae) in their birth canal and it is not known why some babies develop serious Group B Streptococcus (GBS) infection after birth and some do not. There are a number of different ways to screen for GBS in women and there is debate about which women should be offered intrapartum antibiotics.

The National Institute for Health and Clinical Excellence (NICE) and the Royal College of Obstetrics and Gynaecology (RCOG) have published useful guidelines in the UK. There is a NICE guideline 'Antibiotics for the Prevention and Treatment of Early Onset Neonatal Infection' and the recommendations in this chapter are in line with this document.

There are multiple clinical prediction models developed to estimate the risk of neonatal sepsis using a range of predictors, including risk factors, clinical indicators, and/or laboratory tests. An example of such a tool is the Kaiser Permanente neonatal early onset sepsis calculator which is valid for infants from 34 weeks of completed gestational age. However, before the widespread use of these prediction models can be recommended in routine clinical practice in the UK, further studies are needed to validate the use of such tools in UK maternity and neonatal settings.

Sepsis should be a consideration for any baby that is deteriorating, for example in babies identified by Neonatal Early Warning Score (NEWS) chart (Figure 4.1).

Long term outcomes

Neonatal sepsis is a serious condition and untreated infections have a high mortality. If the signs of infection are picked up early and appropriate treatment instituted, the long term outlook is usually good.

Neonatal meningitis is associated with an increased risk of neurodisability and hearing impairment. It is important for these babies to receive neurodevelopmental follow up.

Pathogens

A range of organisms can cause neonatal sepsis. The commonest types of organism are shown in Table 10.1.

Sars-Cov-2 (COVID-19) infection during the coronavirus pandemic, that started in 2019, was uncommon in babies and vertical transmission from the mother, if it occurred at all, was extremely rare.

Table 10.1   Common neonatal pathogens

Micro-organism		Clinical example
Bacteria	Group B Streptococci (GBS)	Commonly cause early onset neonatal sepsis with bacteria acquired from the birth canal. Can also cause late onset neonatal sepsis.
	Gram negative organisms (e.g. Escherichia coli)	Commonly cause early and late onset neonatal sepsis.
	Listeria monocytogenes	Rare in the UK; maternal infection acquired from unpasteurised soft cheese or contaminated pate.
	Chlamydia trachomatis Neisseria gonococcus	Can cause conjunctivitis and serious infection in newborn infants.
	Staphylococcus aureus Coagulase negative Staphylococcus	More commonly found with late sepsis, particularly in those with indwelling central lines.
Viruses	Herpes simplex	Can be transmitted if there are active herpes lesions in the birth canal.
	HIV and Hepatitis B/C	Can be vertically transmitted.
Fungi	Candida albicans	Common cause of nappy rash in babies but can lead to a serious infection especially in the most preterm infants.

Early onset neonatal infection

Early onset neonatal infection is defined as infection occurring during the first 72 h of life. Infection at this time is likely to be caused by organisms acquired in the birth canal. The commonest causative organisms are GBS and E. coli. GBS almost always presents in the first 24 h; after this time other organisms (e.g. E. coli.) are more likely. The introduction of intrapartum antibiotics in mothers known to carry GBS has reduced the incidence of this devastating condition.

Babies that have an increased risk of early onset sepsis can be identified and either observed closely or offered 'risk-based' prophylactic antibiotics.

Risk factors

There are a number of factors that increase the risk of early onset neonatal infection. The presence of these risk factors should be looked for and recorded.

Risk factors for neonatal infection include:
- maternal carriage of GBS (especially if adequate intrapartum antibiotics have not been given)
- maternal GBS bacteruria / urinary tract infection.
- invasive GBS infection in a previous child
- pre-labour rupture of membranes
- intrapartum fever higher than 38°C, if there is suspected or confirmed bacterial infection
- confirmed or suspected chorioamnionitis
- preterm labour
- suspected or confirmed infection in another baby in the case of a multiple pregnancy.

Clinical indicators of early onset infection

The early signs of neonatal infection can be rapid and dramatic or subtle and easily missed.

Early warning scores (see Chapter 4) have been developed to try to identify babies with early signs of infection.

The following clinical indicators can be suggestive of infection:

- the need for cardiopulmonary resuscitation
- tachypnoea and signs of respiratory distress, especially after 4 h of age
- tachycardia
- persistent pulmonary hypertension of the newborn (see Chapter 8)
- signs of shock (see Chapter 8)
- metabolic changes, for example, unexplained acidosis or unstable blood sugar
- temperature instability (either low temperature, high temperature or inability to maintain a stable temperature)
- altered behaviour, tone or handling
- feeding problems.

Red flag risk factors (Table 10.2) should prompt urgent review and intervention.

Table 10.2 Red flag risk factors for neonatal infection

Red flag symptoms for neonatal infection
Maternal IV antibiotics for confirmed or suspected invasive bacterial infection (such as septicaemia) at any time during labour, or in the 24 h periods before and after the birth. (This does not refer to intrapartum antibiotic prophylaxis.)
Suspected or confirmed infection in another baby in the case of a multiple pregnancy
Respiratory distress starting more than 4 h after birth
Seizures
Need for mechanical ventilation in a term baby
Signs of shock

Late onset neonatal infection

Organisms found in the birth canal often cause early onset neonatal infection. In contrast, environmental (nosocomial) organisms often cause late onset infections.

Preterm babies on the neonatal unit are particularly at risk of late onset infection.

The presence of indwelling lines (umbilical lines, long lines and surgically inserted lines) is a significant risk factor, particularly for Staphylococcal infection.

All central lines should be inserted using the strictest aseptic technique. Evidence has shown that obsessive attention to aseptic practices can reduce line infection rates and lead to a significant decrease in morbidity. Some central lines are antibiotic impregnated to try to reduce line infections. The monitoring of Central Line Associated Blood Stream Infections (CLABSI) is a key performance indicator of the quality of neonatal care.

Late onset infections often present with a change in a baby's observations and behaviour. Any change in a baby's status, for instance an increase in the number of episodes of apnoea or bradycardia should prompt a careful review.

Consider antibiotic resistant organisms and unusual infections if the baby fails to respond to treatment. Fungal sepsis can often present insidiously and deep-seated infections such as bacterial endocarditis or osteomyelitis are easily overlooked.

Differential diagnosis

The signs of neonatal sepsis can be non-specific but can also result in rapid deterioration and become life-threatening.

It is worth considering infection as a possible cause in any baby that deteriorates and becomes unwell. It is wise to have a low threshold to consider infection.

Remember that a range of neonatal conditions can look similar to serious infection, for example pneumothorax, necrotising enterocolitis and neonatal respiratory distress syndrome.

Once stabilised, there should be a detailed examination looking for sources of infection.

Managing a baby with signs of neonatal sepsis

Babies with signs of neonatal sepsis should be stabilised using the standard ARNI algorithm and approach (Chapter 1) and Table 10.3.

Table 10.3   The ABCDEF approach to managing Neonatal sepsis

A B	Airway and Breathing	Administer oxygen and increase level of respiratory support to maintain saturations. Consider elective ventilation if there are signs of life-threatening sepsis.
C	Circulation	Babies with life-threatening infection are likely to develop shock. Remember that sepsis can cause vasoconstriction with a delayed capillary refill time but can also present with vasodilatation with distributive shock. Establish early intravenous access, consider fluid boluses and inotropic support as required. Blood products including packed red cells, platelets and fresh frozen plasma (if evidence of coagulopathy) should be considered in line with national guidelines.
D	Disability	Antibiotics should be administered without delay, ideally within the hour of treatment decision. Consider meningitis in any baby, particularly if there are neurological signs (e.g. seizures), once the baby is stable perform a lumbar puncture. Babies with sepsis can present with hypo or hyperglycaemia which needs to be managed appropriately.
E	Exposure and everything else	Consider the source of infection, such as indwelling catheters which may need to be removed to treat the infection adequately. An adequate top to toe examination of the baby, including skin and joints, is needed to look for the source of infection.
F	Family	Parents need to be updated of any changes in baby's condition and treatment. Neonatal infections can be life-threatening and result in a rapid clinical deterioration which can be frightening for parents.

Further investigations

The following tests should be considered when evaluating a baby for sepsis.

Table 10.4 Further investigations for neonatal sepsis

Inflammatory markers	There are a number of inflammatory markers that increase with infection. The most commonly measured marker in neonatal medicine is the C-Reactive Protein (CRP). CRP is made in the liver and is a non-specific marker of infection or inflammation. It takes time for the CRP to rise, and a repeat measurement after 18-24 h can be useful. Babies with overwhelming sepsis can have a normal CRP. The negative predictive value of two normal CRPs is high.
Lactate	Sepsis can cause tissue perfusion problems which cause the lactate to rise.
Blood culture	A positive blood culture is the definitive test for neonatal infection. However, blood cultures are not always positive, even when there is clear evidence of infection. Detection of infection is better with appropriate volumes of blood in the culture bottle. If the baby is not improving repeat cultures should be considered. Remember to check the results of any maternal blood cultures as well as the baby's cultures.
1,3 beta-d-glucan	A highly sensitive but less specific test for neonatal invasive candidiasis in preterm babies.
Lumbar puncture	This should be performed if meningitis is suspected. If raised intracranial pressure may be present e.g. a baby with a subdural haemorrhage, LP would be contraindicated. Some babies do not tolerate lumbar puncture when they are clinically unstable, in this case treat with antibiotics and defer the LP until the baby is more stable. A lumbar puncture should be considered in babies with a positive blood culture.
Urine culture	Urine culture is often not helpful in early onset neonatal sepsis, but urinary tract infection can present as late onset sepsis. The gold standard test is a sterile supra-pubic aspiration of urine. Ultrasound of the bladder can be helpful in guiding this procedure.
Chest X-ray	Congenital pneumonia and ventilator associated chest infection are both common in neonatal intensive care units and a chest X-ray can be a useful diagnostic test especially when there are signs of respiratory distress. Chest X-ray will also exclude pneumothorax as a cause of shock.
Maternal history including results	Thorough review of maternal infection history and results including maternal blood cultures should be undertaken.

Treatment of infection

Prompt antibiotics should be selected to target likely organisms in the first instance. Following initial response, antibiotics can be tailored depending on the results of investigations and clinical progress. The advice of a microbiologist familiar with neonatal infections is invaluable.

Every hospital will have their own guidelines for prescribing antibiotics. These are based on local microbiological surveillance of common organisms and patterns of emerging antimicrobial resistance. Antibiotics for early onset infection should cover both GBS and E. coli. A common antibiotic choice could be benzylpenicillin and gentamicin.

For late onset infection, gram negative and staphylococcal cover is required. If line sepsis from a longline or umbilical catheter is suspected, then removal of the line should be seriously considered.

Anaerobic cover should be considered especially in necrotising enterocolitis.

Antibiotic stewardship is important in neonatal care to minimise unnecessary use of antibiotics. Broad spectrum antibiotics should be used with care; there are an increasing number of multi resistant bacteria and outbreaks of difficult to treat hospital acquired infections are increasingly being reported. Consider the use of prophylactic anti-fungals when using broad spectrum antibiotics, especially in extremely preterm babies.

The duration of antibiotic treatment should be guided by clinical response. The initial minimum duration of antibiotic treatment should be stated at commencement and can be adjusted according to clinical response. In general, a 5 to 7 day course of antibiotics is appropriate for most infections, although longer courses are indicated in serious infections such as meningitis. Some antibiotics (e.g. gentamicin, vancomycin) require therapeutic drug level monitoring.

In a baby who was started on antibiotics largely on the basis of risk factors and who remains clinically well with normal inflammatory markers, it may be appropriate to stop antibiotics once negative cultures have been obtained.

Fungal sepsis can be a serious problem and often requires long course of anti-fungal treatment after liaison with microbiology.

In babies presenting with focal seizures, anti-viral medication should be considered to cover the possibility of Herpes simplex encephalitis.

10: Summary learning

Appropriate timely treatment with antibiotics reduces morbidity and mortality.

Babies at risk of serious infection can often be identified by the presence of risk factors.

The signs of neonatal infection can be subtle and easily overlooked; have a low threshold to investigate and treat for sepsis.

The principles of management follow the standard ARNI algorithm: First stabilise ABC, treat potentially life-threatening features including shock, reassess ABCDEF and implement definitive investigations and treatment.

My key take-home messages from this chapter are:

Further reading

New HV, Stanworth SJ, Gottstein R, Cantwell C, Berryman J, Chalmers EA, Bolton-Maggs PHB, Force BGTT. British Society for Haematology Guidelines on transfusion for fetuses, neonates and older children (Br J Haematol. 2016;175:784-828). Addendum August 2020. Br J Haematol 2020.

National Neonatal Audit Programme (NNAP) 2020 annual report on 2019 data: Royal College of Paediatrics and Child Health On behalf of the NNAP Project Board, November 2020.

Curley A, Stanworth SJ, Willoughby K, Fustolo-Gunnink SF, Venkatesh V, Hudson C, Deary A, Hodge R, Hopkins V, Lopez Santamaria B, Mora A, Llewelyn C, D'Amore A, Khan R, Onland W, Lopriore E, Fijnvandraat K, New H, Clarke P, Watts T, Collaborators PM. Randomized Trial of Platelet-Transfusion Thresholds in Neonates. N Engl J Med 2019; 380: 242-251.

Royal College of Obstetricians and Gynaecologists (2017) Group B streptococcal disease, early-onset (Green-top guideline No. 36). https://www.rcog.org.uk/en/guidelines-research-services/guidelines/gtg36/

National Institute for Health and Clinical Excellence (2020) Neonatal infection: antibiotics for prevention and treatment. London: National Institute for Health and Clinical Excellence. https://www.nice.org.uk/guidance/gid-ng10111/documents/review-questions

National Institute for Health and Clinical Excellence (2017) Intrapartum Care for healthy women and babies CG190. London: National Institute for Health and Clinical Excellence. https://www.nice.org.uk/guidance/cg190

National Institute for Health and Clinical Excellence (2012) Antibiotics for early onset neonatal infection CG149 London: National Institute for Health and Clinical Excellence. www.nice.org.uk/nicemedia/live/13867/60633/60633.pdf

Nuntnarumit P, Pinkaew O, Kitiwanwanich S. Predictive values of serial C-reactive protein in neonatal sepsis. J Med Assoc Thai. 2002 Nov;85 Suppl 4:S1151-8. PMID: 12549789.

Pronovost P, Needham D, Berenholtz S et al. An intervention to decrease catheter related bloodstream infections in the ICU. N Engl J Med. 2006; 355: 2725-2732.

Vergnano S, Sharland M, Kazembe P et al. Neonatal sepsis: an international perspective. Arch Dis Child Fetal Neonatal Ed. 2005; 90: F220-4.

Engle WD, Jackson GL, Sendelbach D et al. Pneumonia in term neonates: laboratory studies and duration of antibiotic therapy. J. Perinatol. 2003: 23: 372-377.

Ruth Gilbert, Michaela Brown, Naomi Rainford, Chloe Donohue, Caroline Fraser, Ajay Sinha, Jon Dorling, Jim Gray, William McGuire, Carrol Gamble, Sam J Oddie, on behalf of the PREVAIL trial team* Antimicrobial-impregnated central venous catheters for prevention of neonatal bloodstream infection (PREVAIL): an open-label, parallel-group, pragmatic, randomised controlled trial. Lancet Child Adolesc Health 2019; 3: 381–90.

Neonatal encephalopathy

In this chapter

Hypoxic ischaemic encephalopathy including clinical management and infomation gathering and sharing

Neurological monitoring

Cerebral function monitoring

Cranial ultrasound scanning

Magnetic resonance imaging

Therapeutic hypothermia

Focal cerebral infarction

Subgaleal haemorrhage

Infection and metabolic disturbances

The learning outcomes will enable you to:

Make the diagnosis of hypoxic ischaemic encephalopathy

Initiate appropriate clinical management

Appreciate the adjuncts used for neurological monitoring

Gain an understanding of when and how to initiate therapeutic hypothermia

Appreciate that there are multiple causes of neonatal encephalopathy

Introduction

Neonatal encephalopathy is a clinical manifestation of disordered neonatal brain function that may present with difficulty in initiating and maintaining respiration, depression of tone and reflexes, subnormal level of consciousness and / or seizures. It is a relatively common clinical condition affecting approximately 1–3.5 per 1000 babies and results in serious consequences for many of the infants including death, cerebral palsy, epilepsy and other significant cognitive, developmental and behavioural problems.

Neonatal encephalopathy may have a number of possible aetiologies including a hypoxic-ischaemic insult, neonatal stroke, infection, metabolic disease and developmental abnormalities.

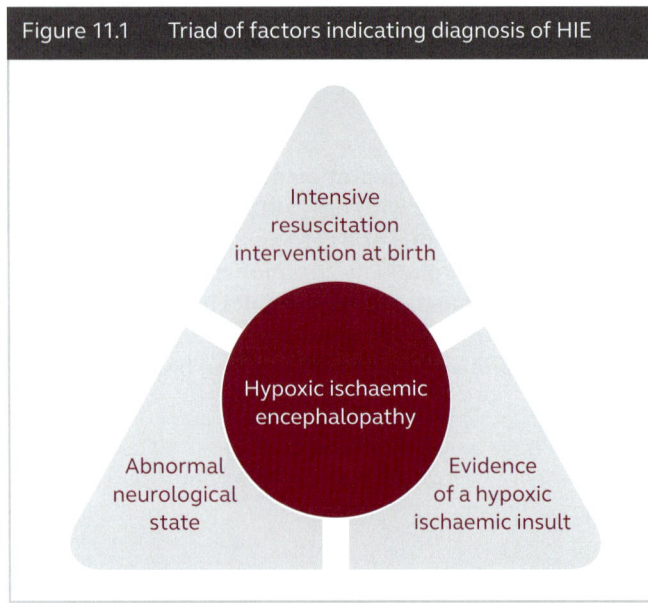

Figure 11.1 Triad of factors indicating diagnosis of HIE

Hypoxic ischaemic encephalopathy (HIE)

Infants usually have a triad of factors (Figure 11.1):

1. intensive resuscitation at birth
2. an abnormal neurological state characterized by abnormal behaviour, tone, reflexes and often seizures
3. evidence of a hypoxic ischaemic insult.

All three components may not be present in every case.

It is difficult to ascertain the timing of a hypoxic ischaemic insult unless a sentinel event has occurred. Defining intrapartum hypoxia-ischaemia as a cord pH ≤ 7.0 is not universally agreed on, as there are reported cases of intrapartum hypoxic ischaemic injury occurring in neonates with cord pH > 7.0. Therefore, there is no single umbilical arterial pH value that clearly distinguishes between cases that have intrapartum hypoxia/ischaemia and those that do not.

Nevertheless, it is generally agreed that the risk for neonatal complications increases as the pH at birth decreases.

Table 11.1 Management of hypoxic ischaemic encephalopathy

On admission to the neonatal unit	Reassess ABCDEF and perform a thorough neurological assessment.
	Consider therapeutic hypothermia.
	Start passive cooling if appropriate. Follow local protocols.
	Insert rectal thermometer at least 3 cm and start continuous rectal temperature monitoring.
	Start mechanical ventilation if poor respiratory drive or repeated seizures.
Cardio-respiratory management	Avoid hypocapnia. Aim for pCO_2 in the normal range during cooling.
	Maintain SaO_2 ≥ 95% to reduce risk of pulmonary hypertension. If giving supplemental oxygen avoid hyperoxia.
	Consider arterial access to monitor blood pressure if mechanical ventilation is required.
	Aim for mean blood pressure (BP) ≥ 40 mmHg.
	A low BP requires assessment. Consider IV 0.9% sodium chloride (10 mL kg^{-1}). Check haematocrit and consider a blood transfusion if clinically hypovolaemic and anaemic.
	Consider inotropes if BP is low despite volume replacement.
	Correct respiratory acidosis by manipulating ventilatory support.
Correction of acidosis	A metabolic acidosis is common and will usually improve if cardiorespiratory stability is maintained. If a severe metabolic acidosis persists consider treating with intravenous sodium bicarbonate.
	Hypoglycaemia can be a serious complicating factor in HIE. Monitor plasma glucose closely and adjust glucose intake accordingly.
Fluid balance/metabolic management	Oliguria/anuria is common following moderate/severe HIE, start initial maintenance fluids at 40–60 mL kg day^{-1} this minimise cerebral oedema electrolyte imbalances.
	Avoid hypoglycaemia.
	Watch for syndrome of inappropriate excretion of anti-diuretic hormone (SIADH) and avoid severe hyponatraemia.
	Monitor urinary output and observe for urinary retention. Bladder catheterisation may be useful.
	Avoid fluid overload during oliguria and avoid hypovolaemia once diuresis starts.
	Consider low dose dopamine (2.5–5 micrograms kg $mins^{-1}$) or fluid challenge (10 mL kg 0.9% sodium chloride IV over 30 min) in incipient renal failure.
	Watch for accumulation of nephrotoxic drugs e.g. gentamicin and adjust doses accordingly.
	Consider electrolyte additives or parenteral nutrition after 24–48 h when electrolytes/renal function stable.
Monitoring for multiorgan failure	Monitor haematological, clotting, biochemical, renal and hepatic function parameters.

Equally the use of other parameters including a low Apgar score, the presence of meconium stained liquor, fetal heart rate abnormalities on cardiotocograph are all not specific or sensitive enough for the diagnosis of intrapartum hypoxia on their own.

Although therapeutic hypothermia improves outcomes in term infants with moderate HIE and is now the standard of care, meticulous medical and nursing intensive care, is also critical. The includes: management of multiorgan dysfunction, obtaining and documenting detailed clinical information and performing appropriate investigations to confirm a diagnosis. This will help direct care and inform counselling and support to the family.

Clinical management on the neonatal unit

The initial management (Table 11.1) of infants with HIE following admission to the neonatal unit consists of standard neonatal intensive care measures, continuous core temperature monitoring and initiation of therapeutic hypothermia if appropriate. In some cases, passive cooling may have been commenced on labour ward, however, this should only be started once the baby has been stabilised and continuous core temperature monitoring is in place. Neurological monitoring by regular clinical examination, continuous EEG or amplitude integrated EEG (aEEG) and cranial ultrasound examination is recommended.

Clinical management will depend on the severity of encephalopathy. Infants with mild encephalopathy at about 6 hours of age are likely to make a rapid recovery but may occasionally deteriorate and have brief seizures. Observation (preferably including aEEG) for at least 24 h should be considered. These infants may be enterally fed according to local protocols. More severely affected infants will require closer monitoring and enteral feeding can be cautiously introduced once the initial biochemical and metabolic disturbance are corrected, usually after about 24 h, even if the infant is receiving therapeutic hypothermia.

Information gathering and documentation

Many cases present unexpectedly, and the focus following birth is on clinical management of both baby and mother; consequently, communication and information sharing between obstetric and neonatal teams may be suboptimal. However, it is important to obtain a detailed structured clinical history to identify risk factors for HIE, evidence of alternative diagnoses and comorbidities. This information needs to be carefully documented so that it is readily available to multidisciplinary teams involved in the short and long term clinical management. It is important to remember that medicolegal scrutiny of possible HIE is common; documentation should be clear, contemporaneous and record fact rather than assumption.

Neurological monitoring

Regular neurological assessment (Table 11.2) is necessary to determine the severity of encephalopathy, detect deterioration and complications, to assess the response to treatments such as anticonvulsant therapy and to assess likely neurological outcome which is critical for planning further clinical management.

Table 11.2 Neurological monitoring

The clinical features of HIE evolve over a period of days. Perform daily neurological examinations and document clinical state and responsiveness.
Perform continuous aEEG according to local protocols.
Monitor for seizures: correlate subtle signs such as lip smacking, head turning, eye turning, bradycardias and apnoeas with the aEEG. Subclinical seizures may be apparent on aEEG.
Treat clinical and subclinical seizures according to local protocols.
Widely used first line treatment is: Phenobarbitone 20 mg kg^{-1} loading dose, repeating a second loading dose 10–20 mg kg^{-1} if seizure control is not achieved.
Options for 2nd and 3rd line anticonvulsants, listed alphabetically include either: − Levetiracetam 20 mg kg^{-1} over 20 min that may be repeated to a maximum total dose of 60 mg kg^{-1} − *Lidocaine 2 mg kg^{-1} loading over 10 min then 4–6 mg kg h^{-1} for maximum of 24 h − Midazolam 60 micrograms kg h^{-1} (max 300 micrograms kg h^{-1}) − *Phenytoin 20 mg kg^{-1} over 30 min − *Lidocaine and phenytoin should not be given together in view of risk of precipitating arrhythmias − While seizures are common in HIE, unremitting seizure activity should lead to urgent consideration of other causes of epileptic encephalopathy, including consideration of a trial of pyridoxine.
Cooling affects the pharmacokinetics of many anticonvulsants and care should be taken to avoid accumulation, particularly when using infusions.
Perform cranial ultrasound scans and measure cerebral flow velocities and calculate resistive index according to local protocols.
Perform MRI according to local protocols. The optimal timing for a scan is 5–15 days after birth.

Several clinical neonatal neurological examination methods have been described which help standardise the assessment of HIE and are part of the criteria for starting therapeutic hypothermia e.g. modified Sarnat staging (Table 11.3) or Thompson scores. Assessment may be complicated by anticonvulsant therapies, muscle relaxing agents and co-morbidities. Seizures are common in the context of hypoxic-ischaemic encephalopathy but also have other causes.

Investigation of neonatal seizures

First line investigations for seizures

- Consider blood glucose, serum calcium, magnesium, blood gas, urea and electrolytes, blood culture.
- Correct blood glucose or electrolyte abnormalities.
- Consider cerebral function monitoring.

Second line investigations for seizures

- Consider lumbar puncture (if not contraindicated), virology studies, congenital infection screen, cranial ultrasound, MRI brain, toxicology screen.
- Start anticonvulsants for persistent or prolonged seizures.
- Consideration of a trial of pyridoxine in very resistant seizures.

Cerebral function monitoring (CFM)

Continuous cerebral function monitoring (Figure 11.3) using an amplitude integrated electroencephalogram (aEEG) is good practice and is increasing being performed in local neonatal units and special care centres, prior to transfer to a cooling centre. It is easy and quick to apply, the patterns are relatively simple to analyse and correlate well with both standard EEG, MRI findings and neurological outcome. Severely abnormal patterns such as burst suppression or low voltage patterns persisting for more than about 24 h after birth are associated with a poor neurodevelopmental outcome in about 70% of infants, even in infants treated with hypothermia. Abnormal patterns that normalise over about 24 h are associated with a better prognosis.

Interpretation

Two things are taken into account, the upper and lower voltage margins of the aEEG trace and the pattern of the trace. These are illustrated in Figures 11.4-11.7.

Table 11.3   Modified Sarnat Score

Domain	Stage 1	Stage 2	Stage 3
Seizures	None	Common focal or multifocal seizures	Uncommon (excluding decerebration) Or frequent seizures
Level of consciousness	Normal Hyperalert	Lethargic Decreased activity in an infant who is aroused and responsive Can be irritable to external stimuli	Stuperose/ comatose Not able to rouse and unresponsive to external stimuli
Spontaneous activity when awake or aroused	Active Vigorous, does not stay in one position	Less than active Not vigorous	No activity whatsoever
Posture	Moving around and does not maintain any position	Distal flexion Complete extension or frog legged posture	Decerebrate with or without stimulation (all extremities extended)
Tone	Normal- resists passive motion Hypertonic, jittery	Hypotonic or floppy, either focal or general	Completely flaccid
Primitive reflexes	Vigorously sucks finger or ET tube Normal Moro reflex	Suck: weak Moro: incomplete	Suck: completely absent Moro: completely absent
Autonomic system	Pupils: normal size Reactive to light Heart rate: normal > 100 Respirations normal	Pupils constricted < 3mm but react to light Heart rate: bradycardia (< 100 variable up to 120) Respirations: periodic irregular breathing effort	Pupils: fixed dilated, skew gaze not reactive to light Heart rate: variable, inconsistent rate, irregular may be bradycardia. Respirations: completely apnoeic requiring positive pressure ventilation
Outcome	Normal	25% abnormal with cerebral palsy	Abnormal / death in 75%

The normal amplitude (Figure 11.4)

The upper margin of band aEEG activity > 10μV AND the lower margin > 5 μV. Sleep wave cycling can also be seen as the band of activity narrows during periods of sleep. This may also be seen with mild encephalopathy.

Moderately abnormal amplitude (Figure 11.5)

The upper margin of band aEEG activity > 10μV AND the lower margin < 5 μV. This makes the band broader.

Severely abnormal amplitude (Figure 11.6)

The upper margin of band aEEG activity < 10μV AND the lower margin < 5 μV. This makes the band narrower.

Seizures (Figure 11.7)

A rapid rise in baseline often showing a saw toothed pattern.

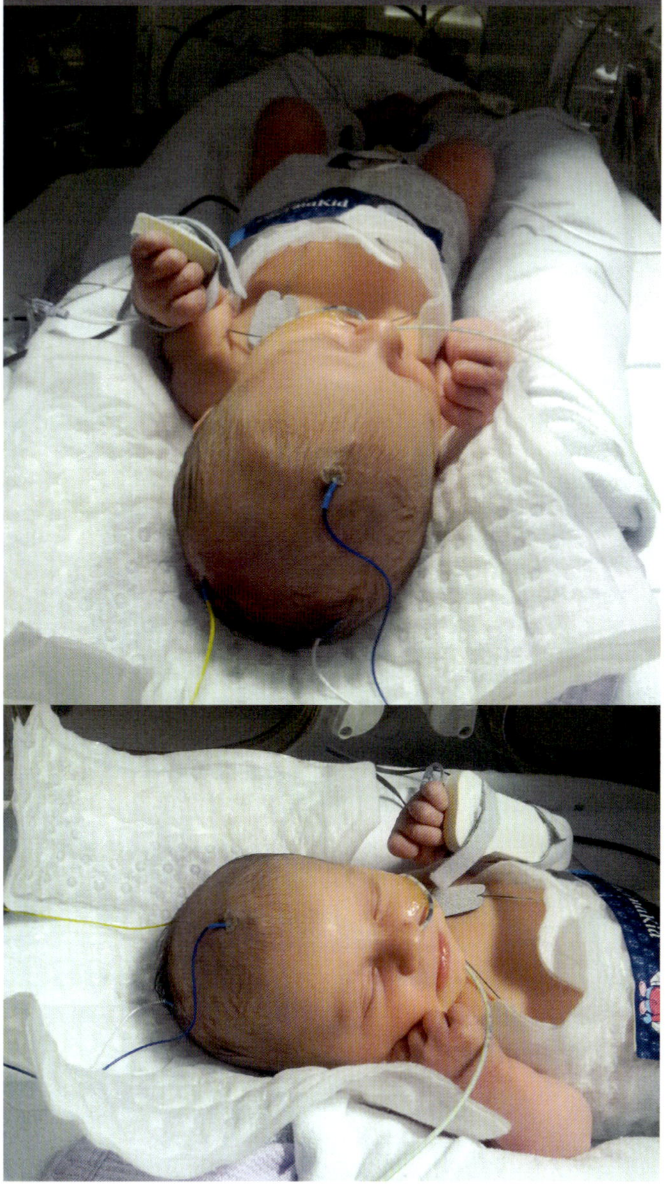

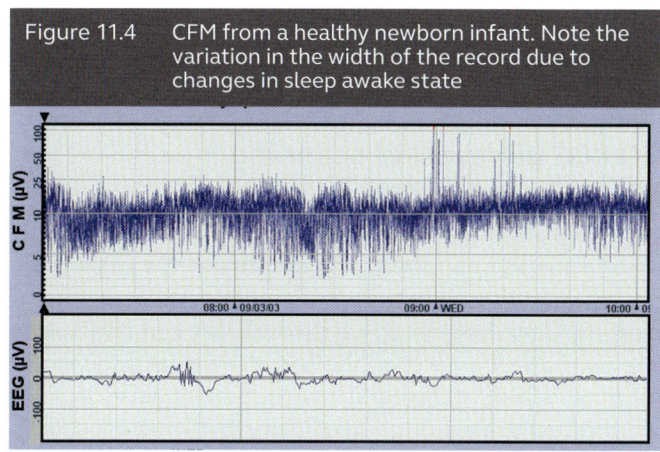

Figure 11.4 CFM from a healthy newborn infant. Note the variation in the width of the record due to changes in sleep awake state

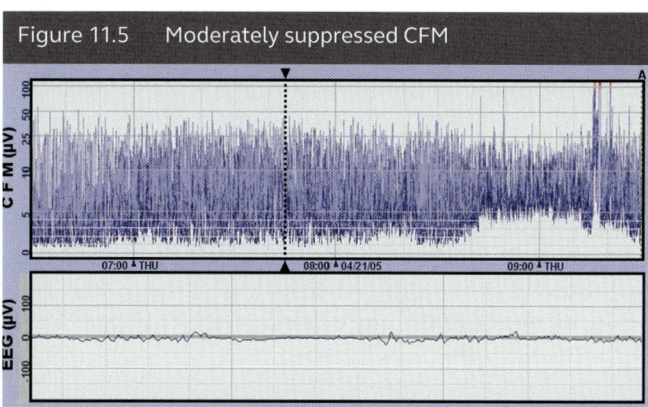

Figure 11.5 Moderately suppressed CFM

Figure 11.3 Term baby undergoing therapeutic hypothermia with CFM needles in situ

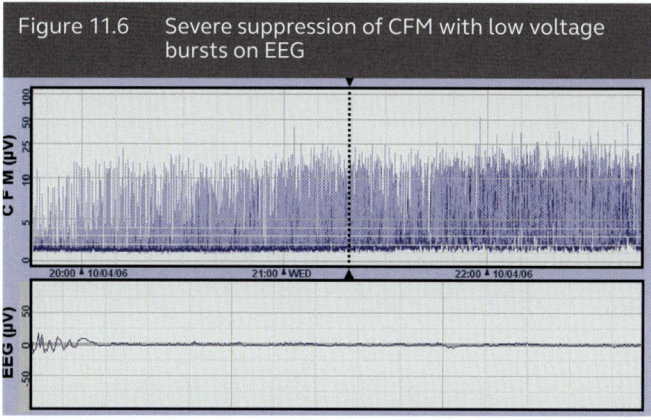

Figure 11.6 Severe suppression of CFM with low voltage bursts on EEG

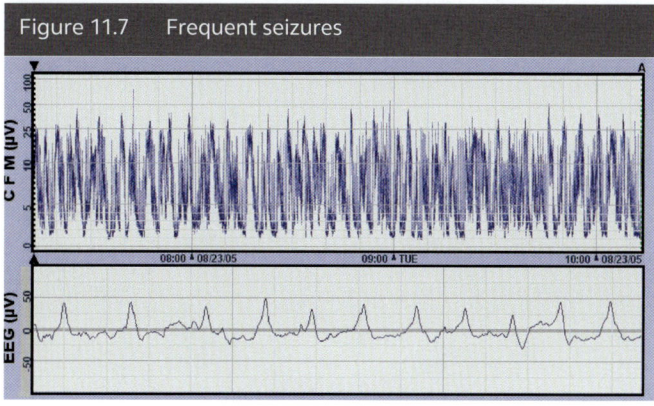

Figure 11.7 Frequent seizures

Cranial ultrasound scanning

Cranial ultrasound scanning is helpful to exclude structural abnormality which might suggest metabolic or other diagnoses, detect calcification and cysts suggestive of viral infection and detect atrophy suggestive of long standing damage. It may also identify cerebral haemorrhage or infarction. An early cranial ultrasound may not identify all cerebral injuries. Sequential observation of the evolution of injury following a recent hypoxic ischaemic insult at birth can be helpful. This helps in defining the pattern of injury and timing its onset. Features of cerebral oedema may be present initially with generalised increased echodensity and compressed ventricles. More severe cases may have increased echodensity in the basal ganglia.

Cerebral Doppler ultrasound measurements can help to guide prognosis. There should always be forward flow in the cerebral vessels throughout the cardiac cycle and the height of the peak systolic velocity is generally about 3–4 times the height of the end diastolic velocity (Figure 11.7).

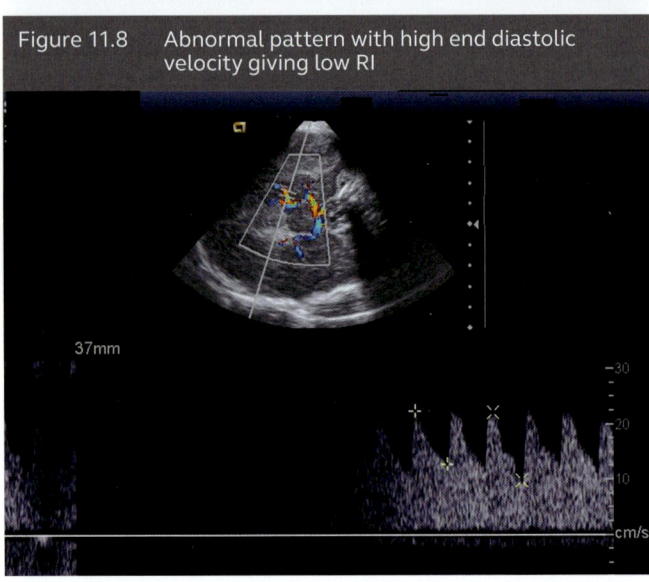

Figure 11.7   Normal cerebral doppler pattern

Figure 11.8   Abnormal pattern with high end diastolic velocity giving low RI

The measurement of the blood flow velocity from the anterior or middle cerebral arteries can be used to derive a resistive index (RI):

RI = (peak systolic velocity – end diastolic velocity) divided by peak systolic velocity

The **normal range** after the first few hours of life is 0.65–0.85.

Abnormal is < 0.55 (Figure 11.8) on 2 to 3 occasions within 24–72 h from birth.

This suggests a loss of normal vasoreactivity secondary to a hypoxic ischaemic insult and is predictive for a poor neurological outcome or death providing that at the time of the measurement the blood pressure and arterial pCO_2 are in the normal range and the baby is not having seizures. Measurement of resistive index can be subject to inter-operator error.

Magnetic resonance imaging

Magnetic resonance imaging (MRI) may provide useful information for prognostication or show specific patterns of abnormality that may suggest diagnoses other than HIE (Figure 11.9). Some cranial MRI scans within 24 h of birth may appear normal or have findings predominantly associated with brain swelling, such as loss of extracerebral space, sulcal markings and slit like anterior horns of the lateral ventricles.

Scans obtained later in the first week may show severe injury. It is for this reason that the recommended time for an MRI is between 5–15 days. The most common pattern of severe acute injury observed is damage to the basal ganglia, thalami and cortex. The appearances of the posterior limb of the internal capsule (PLIC) and the involvement of the cortex are important in counselling parents regarding the likely long term prognosis (Figure 11.9).

Therapeutic hypothermia

Unless you have decided to implement hypothermia, take active steps to maintain the temperature of the newly born infant between 36.5°C and 37.5°C from birth to admission and throughout stabilisation. For each 1°C decrease in admission temperature below this range there is an associated relative increase in mortality by 28%.

However, clinical studies have shown that a 3–4°C reduction of brain and body temperature (Figure 11.10a) following hypoxic ischaemic insult reduces cerebral injury and protects cerebral function, primarily by reducing cerebral metabolic activity and apoptotic cell death. The precise mechanism of neural rescue is uncertain

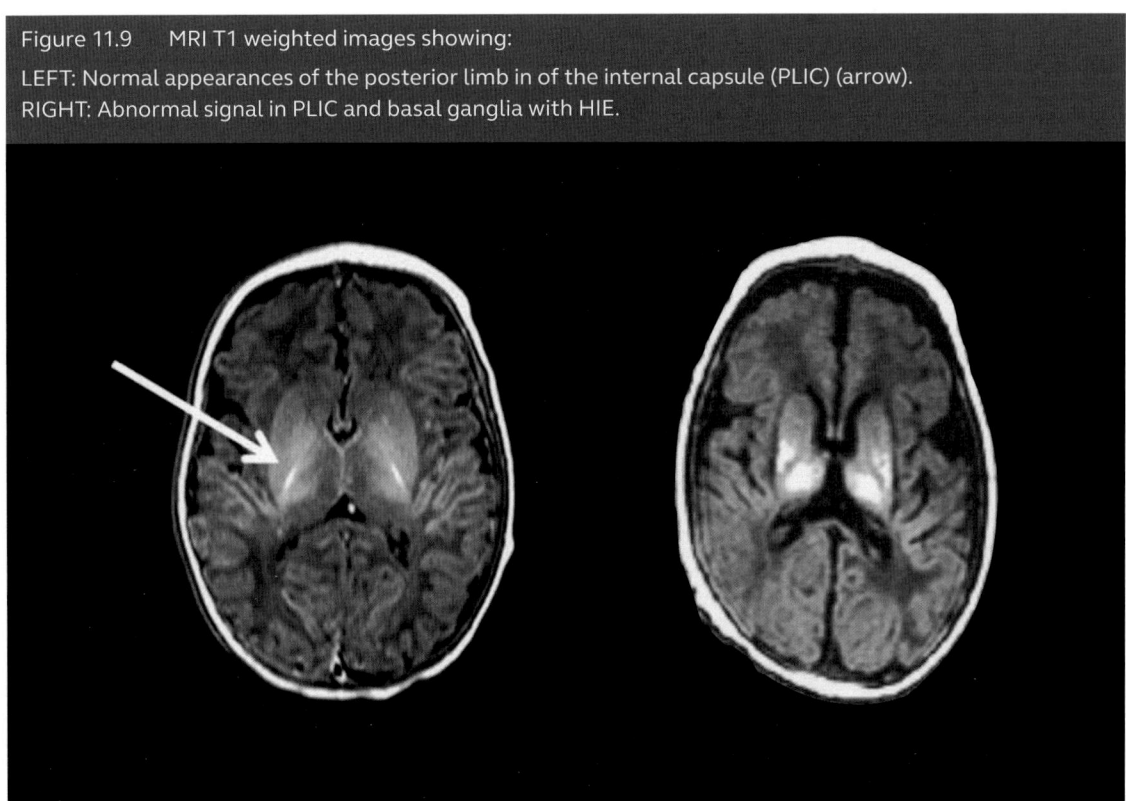

Figure 11.9 MRI T1 weighted images showing:
LEFT: Normal appearances of the posterior limb in of the internal capsule (PLIC) (arrow).
RIGHT: Abnormal signal in PLIC and basal ganglia with HIE.

but may be related to the critical relationship between temperature and metabolic rate: for every 1°c lowering of core temperature, cerebral metabolism is reduced by approximately 7%, with consequently a lower glucose and oxygen demand. Moderate hypothermia is associated with a reduction in free radicals and glutamate levels, protecting mitochondrial function and maintaining cerebral high energy phosphate levels.

Term or near-term infants, with evolving moderate to severe hypoxic-ischaemic encephalopathy, should be treated with therapeutic hypothermia (Figure 11.10a and 11.10b). Cooling should be initiated and conducted under clearly defined protocols and should only commence after airway, breathing and circulation priorities have been addressed. Early identification and assessment for evidence of hypoxic ischaemic encephalopathy and seizures is crucial, as therapeutic hypothermia should be commenced within 6 h and continued for 72 h. Passive cooling should be commenced in a controlled way after resuscitation is completed if the perinatal history is strongly suggestive of hypoxic ischaemic encephalopathy. Once the decision to continue with cooling is made, active cooling can be commenced in an appropriate centre. If available, amplitude integrated EEG aids clinical assessment especially in infants with borderline moderate encephalopathy, and when clinical seizures are suspected.

Treatment criteria for cooling

A. Infants ≥ 36 completed weeks gestation admitted to the neonatal unit with at least one of the following:

- Apgar score of ≤ 5 at 10 min after birth
- Continued need for resuscitation, including tracheal or mask ventilation, at 10 min after birth
- Acidosis within 60 min of birth (defined as any occurrence of umbilical cord, arterial or capillary pH < 7.0)
- Base Deficit ≥ 16 mmol L^{-1} in umbilical cord or any blood sample (arterial, venous or capillary) within 60 min of birth.

Infants that meet criteria A should be assessed for whether they meet the neurological abnormality entry criteria (B):

B. Seizures or moderate to severe encephalopathy, consisting of:

- Altered state of consciousness (reduced or absent response to stimulation) and
- Abnormal tone (focal or general hypotonia, or flaccid) and
- Abnormal primitive reflexes (weak or absent suck or Moro response).

Infants who meet criteria A and B may be considered for treatment with cooling.

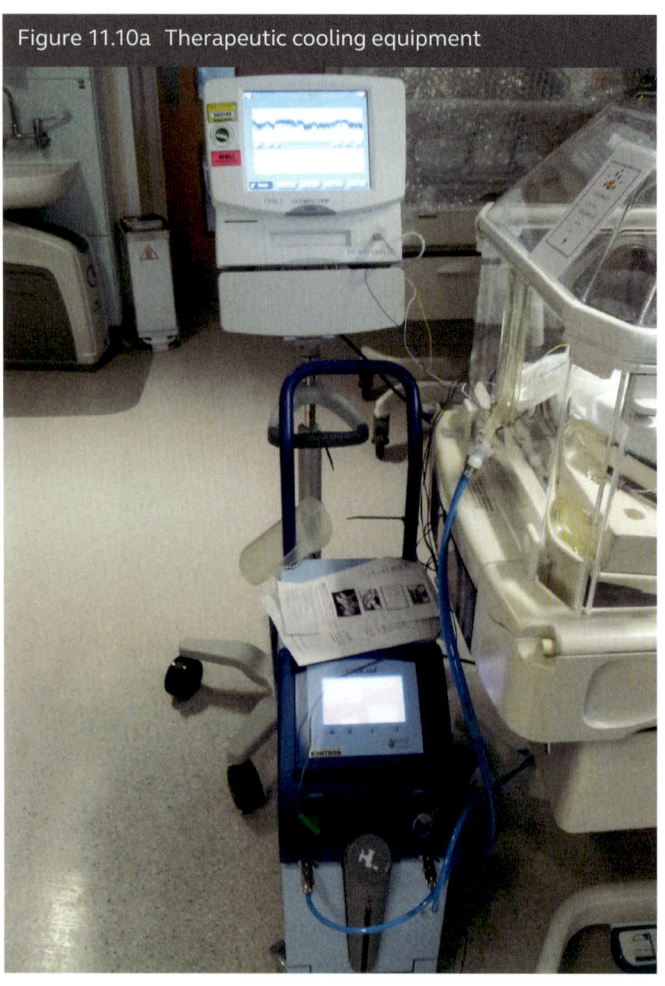

Figure 11.10a Therapeutic cooling equipment

The optimal rate of re-warming is not clear but clinical deterioration during rewarming has been reported in adult studies and there is anecdotal experience of worsening of the amplitude integrated EEG and recurrence of seizures in the re-warming phase. For these reasons current advice is to re-warm gradually over about 12 h.

Prognosis

A major challenge in the clinical care of infants with severe hypoxic ischaemic encephalopathy is the assessment of prognosis. It is often difficult to assess the therapeutic response to hypothermia during the first few days after birth, sometimes because of morphine infusions or the sedative effects of anticonvulsants which can hinder clinical assessment.

The prognosis becomes increasingly poor the longer the infant remains in a severe encephalopathic state (Stage 3 encephalopathy) and the longer the aEEG/EEG remains severely suppressed (EEG voltage extremely low or absent). Some severely affected infants have a partial recovery during the first 72 h after birth but the level of encephalopathy persists at an intermediate stage 2/3, with the aEEG/EEG remaining moderately or severely abnormal (burst suppression pattern of the EEG predominating).

The occurrence of severe basal ganglia and thalami signal abnormalities usually together with moderate/severe white matter and cortical changes on MRI, predicts a very poor prognosis. This may include spastic quadriplegia,

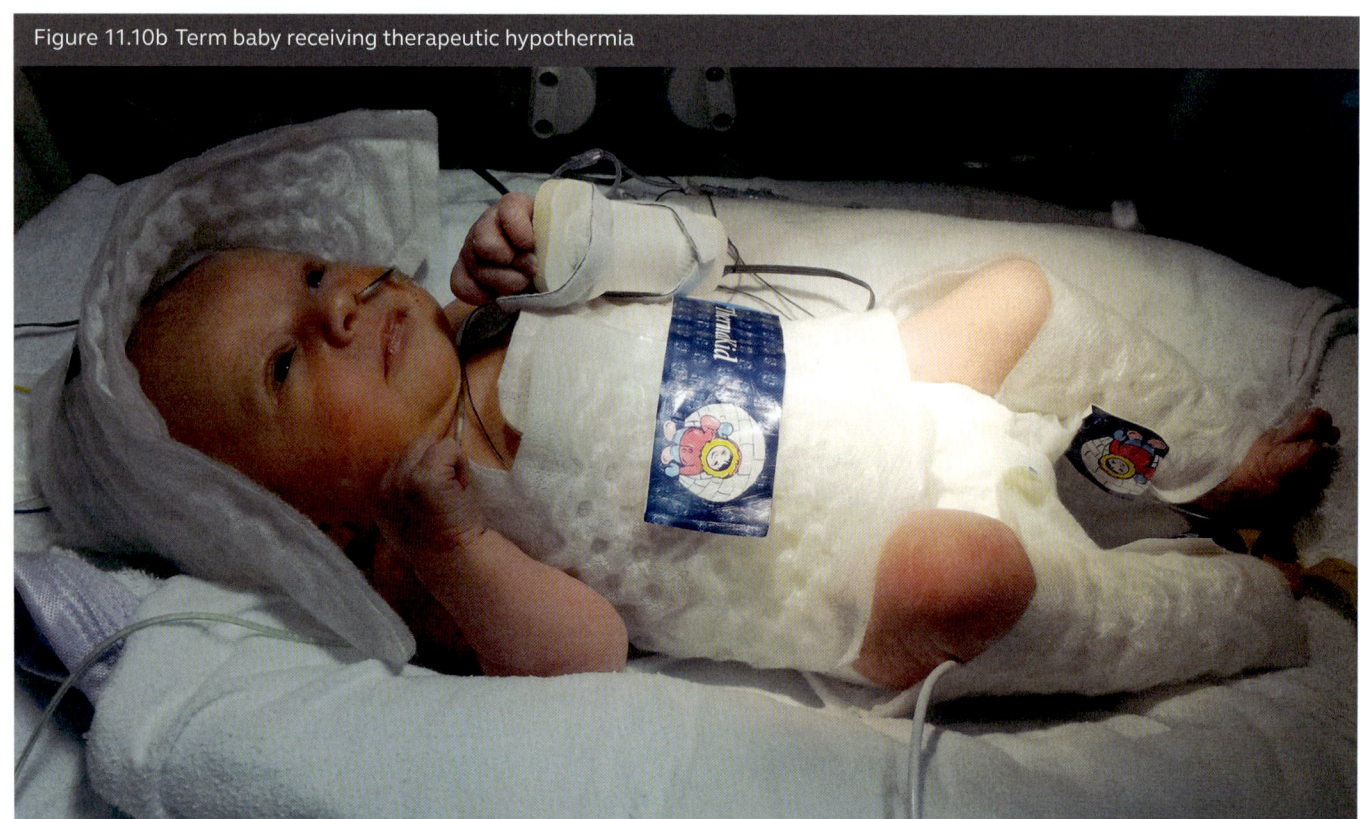

Figure 11.10b Term baby receiving therapeutic hypothermia

microcephaly, feeding problems, visual and other communicative difficulties even in infants treated with hypothermia.

Rapid improvement in neurological signs and early establishment of oral feeding are associated with a more favourable prognosis.

Key treatment points during therapeutic hypothermia

- Early identification and assessment of infants for evidence of HIE is essential.
- Commence passive cooling after resuscitation if perinatal history is strongly suggestive of HIE. Continuous core temperature monitoring must be in place (Figure 11.10 a/b).
- Commence active cooling in an appropriate centre once treatment criteria are met. Active cooling in transport is recommended.
- Target temperature of 33–34°C.
- Continuous aEEG, vital signs and rectal temperature monitoring.
- Daily neurological assessment.
- Cranial ultrasound scans according to local protocol.
- Provide adequate sedation.
- Use local protocol for management of seizures.
- After 72 h of induced hypothermia re-warming should be carried out over 12 h.

Focal cerebral infarction

Neonatal stroke is an area of damaged cerebral tissue which may be either ischaemic or haemorrhagic in origin. Arterial ischaemic strokes, secondary to thrombosis or embolism, are the most common type of neonatal stroke with the left middle cerebral artery being the most commonly involved vessel. The incidence is reported as 1 in 2300–4000 deliveries and is the diagnosis in 10–15% of neonates with seizures. It accounts for approximately 30% of childhood hemiplegia.

Newborn infants who have had a cerebral infarction do not usually require significant resuscitation, although labour and delivery are often complicated. Apgar scores and cord gases are often within normal limits. They may have been initially well on the postnatal wards with their mother prior to presenting with seizures or apnoeas, hypotonia, episodes of duskiness, irritability or poor feeding. 90% of cases present within 3 days of delivery.

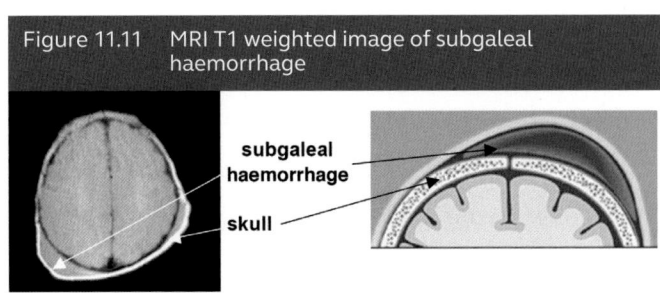

Figure 11.11 MRI T1 weighted image of subgaleal haemorrhage

Subgaleal haemorrhage

Although rare, subgaleal haemorrhages (Figure 11.11) potentially life threatening and are most often associated with vacuum extraction or forceps delivery. The bleeding is caused by the rupture of emissary veins which connect the dural sinuses and scalp veins. Large volumes of blood may accumulate in the loose connective tissue below the subaponeurotic membrane very quickly leading to hypovolaemia, multiorgan failure and even death if not recognised. The first signs may be of pallor or hypovolaemic shock. The head circumference increases rapidly and the soft tissue swelling crosses the suture lines. Rapid ABC assessment, diagnosis, intensive care and blood product support is essential.

Infection and metabolic disturbances

Meningitis, hypoglycaemia and electrolyte disturbance must always be considered in a baby presenting with neonatal encephalopathy or seizures. Investigations to exclude these are routinely performed in babies presenting with neonatal encephalopathy but further discussion on these is beyond the remit of this chapter.

11: Summary learning

Neonatal encephalopathy is relatively common and can result in significant morbidity or mortality.

Neonatal encephalopathy has a range of different causes although a hypoxic ischaemic injury is the commonest.

Apnoeas in a term baby are frequently due to seizures.

Meticulous monitoring and documentation is required.

My key take-home messages from this chapter are:

Further reading

Archer LN, Levene Ml, Evans DH. Cerebral artery Doppler ultrasonography for prediction of outcome after perinatal asphyxia. Lancet 1986; 2: 1116-1118.

Azzopardi DV, Strohm B, Edwards AD, et al. Moderate hypothermia to treat perinatal asphyxia! encephalopathy. N Engl J Med 2009; 361: 1349-358.

Azzopardi D. Clinical management of the baby with hypoxic ischaemic encephalopathy. Early Human Development 201 0; 86: 345-350.

BAPM. Therapeutic Hypothermia for Neonatal Encephalopathy. A Framework for Practice. November 2020

Edwards AD, Brocklehurst P, Gunn AJ, et al. Neurological outcomes at 18 months of age after moderate hypothermia for perinatal hypoxic ischaemic encephalopathy: synthesis and meta-analysis of trial data. BMJ 201 0; 340: c363.

Eken P, Toet MC, Groenendaal F, et al. Predictive value of early neuroimaging, pulsed Doppler and neurophysiology in full term infants with hypoxicischaemic encephalopathy. Arch Dis Child Fetal Neonatal Ed. 1995; 73: F75-80.

Gale C, Statnikov Y, Jawad S, Uthaya SN, Modi N, Brain Injuries expert working g. Neonatal brain injuries in England: population-based incidence derived from routinely recorded clinical data held in the National Neonatal Research Database. Archives of disease in childhood Fetal and neonatal edition. 2018;103(4):F301-F6.

Gluckman PD, Wyatt JS, Azzopardi D, al. Selective head cooling with mild systemic hypothermia after neonatal encephalopathy: multicentre randomised trial. Lancet 2005; 365: 663-670.

Graham EM, Ruis KA, Hartman AL, et al. A systematic review of the role of intrapartum hypoxia-ischemia in the causation of neonatal encephalopathy. Am J Obstet Gynecol 2008;199(6):587-95.

Kumar S, Paterson-Brown S. Obstetric aspects of hypoxic ischemic encephalopathy Early Human Development 201 0; 86: 339-344.

Rutherford M, Malamateniou C, McGuinness A, et al. Magnetic resonance imaging in hypoxic-ischaemic encephalopathy. Early Human Development 2010; 86: 351-360.

Rutherford MA, Ramenghi LA, Cowan FM. Neonatal stroke. Arch Dis Fetal Neonatal Ed. 2012; 97: F377-384.

Sarnat HB, Sarna! MS. Neonatal encephalopathy following fetal distress. A clinical and electroencephalographic study. Arch Neural 1976; 33: 696-705.

Shankaran S, Laptook AR, Ehrenkranz RA, et al. Whole body hypothermia for neonates with hypoxic-ischemic encephalopathy. N Engl J Med 2005; 353:

RCOG. Each Baby Counts progress report 2018.

Toet MC, van Rooij LG, de Vries LS. The use of amplitude integrated electroencephalography for assessing neonatal neurologic injury. Clin Perinatal. 2008;35(4): 665-78.

Thompson CM, Puterman AS, Linley LL, et al. The value of a scoring system for hypoxic ischaemic encephalopathy in predicting neurodevelopmental outcome. Acta Paediatr 1997; 86: 757-61.

UK TOBY Cooling Register Clinician's Handbook Version 4, May 2010 Battin M, Bennet L, Gunn AJ. Rebound seizures during rewarming. Pediatrics 2004;114(5):1369.

Van den Broek MPH, Rademaker CNA, van Straaten HLM et al. Anticonvulsant treatment of asphyxiated newborns under hypotherma with lidocaine: efficacy, safety and dosing. Arch Dis Child Fetal Neonatal Ed. 2013: 98: F341-5.

Unexpected problems in the term infant

In this chapter

Sudden unexpected postnatal ward collapse (SUPC)

Approach to assessment, resuscitation, management and investigation of SUPC

When to consider stopping resuscitation

Considerations post resuscitation

Communication with parents

Treatment considerations of some specific aetiologies of SUPC

The learning outcomes will enable you to:

Be able to recognise, investigate and manage unexpected problems in the term infant

Develop an approach to rapid assessment, resuscitation, management and investigation of the collapsed infant

Introduction

Apparently healthy infants on the postnatal ward can rarely suffer sudden deterioration or collapse.

As shown below, in many babies who suffer a sudden unexpected postnatal collapse, the cause remains unexplained. However, of those in whom a diagnosis is made, bacterial infection and congenital abnormalities (particularly cardiac) are most frequently seen (see Figure 12.1). Persistent pulmonary hypertension of the newborn (PPHN) can be associated with postnatal ward collapse but is often secondary to the underlying cause.

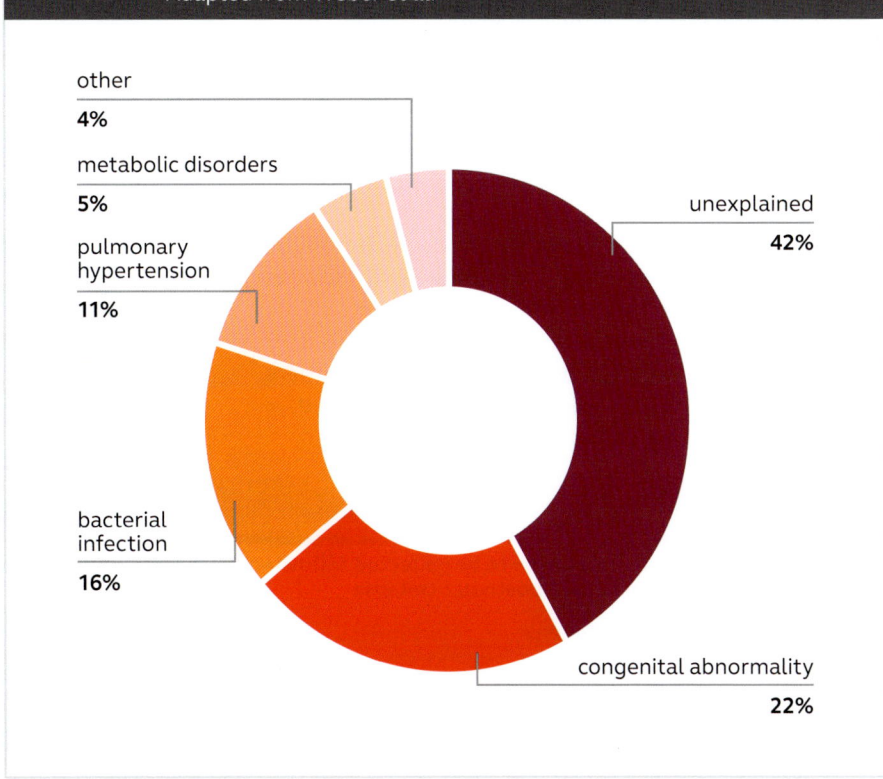

Figure 12.1 Causes of death from a series of 55 sudden unexpected neonatal deaths undergoing post mortem examination. Adapted from Weber et al.

Sudden unexpected postnatal collapse (SUPC)

An infant who suffers a 'Sudden Unexpected Postnatal Collapse' includes any term or near term (> 35 weeks gestation) infant who:

- is well at birth (normal 5 minute Apgar score and deemed well enough to have routine postnatal care) and,
- collapses within the first seven days of life and,
- either dies, goes onto require intensive care or develops an encephalopathy.

SUPC is rare with a reported incidence of about 1 in 20 000 live births. It is a serious and potentially devastating event resulting in death in up to 30% of affected infants. Many of the survivors will have significant long term neurodevelopmental sequelae.

There are differences between SUPC and Sudden Unexpected Death in Infancy (SUDI). The majority of SUDI cases occur outside the hospital setting and by definition do not include the survivors of a sudden postnatal collapse.

Infants with SUPC have a higher incidence of identifiable underlying pathological conditions unlike SUDI. However, like SUDI a significant proportion of SUPC infants also collapse following accidental suffocation. This is associated with prone positioning, primiparous mothers, breast feeding and co-sleeping where mother is tired, under the influence of drugs or alcohol.

Approach to assessment, resuscitation, management and investigation

In any acute life-threatening event, the approach to the collapsed infant should follow the ARNI approach to assessment and treatment (Table 12.1).

The aim of the initial treatment is to keep the patient alive and hopefully achieve some clinical improvement allowing time to make a diagnosis and plan definitive care. Following the ARNI algorithm (see Chapter 1) will facilitate the early management.

Remember to investigate the history or circumstances of the collapse as this may assist in making a diagnosis.

Key treatment points

- Assess ABCDEF.
- Treat potentially life-threatening conditions immediately before moving on.
- Initial resuscitation and stabilisation is aimed at sustaining life and supporting organ systems and hopefully achieving some improvement to allow time to make a diagnosis and plan definitive care.

Following initial assessment and management of potentially life-threatening conditions, the baby should be reassessed and attention turned to making a diagnosis and establishing definitive care.

This secondary assessment should include additional history (Table 12.2); further investigations (Table 12.3) will be guided by progress and history.

Table 12.2 Additional information to be collected following sudden unexpected postnatal collapse

Parental medical history	Medications
Parental substance misuse	Recreational drugs, alcohol
Family history	Recurrent miscarriage or neonatal death
Obstetric history	Recent illnesses, antenatal scan results (growth, liquor volume, anomalies, dopplers)
Labour and birth history	Maternal medications, risk of sepsis, suspected asphyxia (cord/scalp pH, CTG), meconium, condition at birth
Postnatal progress until collapse	Exact circumstances surrounding collapse, including position of baby and feeding

Table 12.3 Additional investigations in sudden unexpected postnatal collapse

In addition to first line investigations consider the following:	Renal and liver function tests
	Coagulation screen
	Calcium, magnesium
	Ammonia, lactate, blood gas
	Serum for viral studies
	Lithium heparin samples for later metabolic/endocrine investigations
	Consider maternal Kleihauer, virology, vaginal swabs
	The placenta should be sent for histopathological examination if it is available
	Blood for DNA storage
	Collect blood on a standard blood spot test paper for acyl carnitine profile
	Imaging investigations
	Cardiac investigations e.g. ECG, echocardiogram

Table 12.1 Specific assessments and actions in the initial ABCDEF approach in sudden unexpected postnatal collapse

Assessment		Information sought	Possible resultant actions
A	Airway patency	Look for signs of obstruction ('see saw' breathing, severe intercostal/subcostal recession) No breath sounds in complete obstruction An unconscious infant may not maintain airway patency	Call for expert help immediately Place baby's head in neutral position Jaw thrust Suction (if indicated) Insert a laryngeal mask or oropharyngeal airway Intubate if required Give oxygen Reassess
B	Breathing adequacy	Look for potentially life-threatening conditions (apnoea/pneumothorax) Is the baby breathing? Look, listen and feel for signs of respiratory distress Look for cyanosis Measure the respiratory rate Are the breath sounds equal? Measure the oxygen saturations	Administer oxygen Support breathing with bag valve mask ventilation and consider intubation Consider cold light examination, needle aspiration or chest drain insertion if pneumothorax suspected
C	Circulation adequacy	Assess for hypovolaemia: Are the peripheries cold? What is the capillary refill time? Is the infant tachycardic (heart rate > 150)? Assess the pulses (reduced in shock or critically obstructed systemic circulation e.g. aortic stenosis, reduced femoral pulses in coarctation of the aorta). Are there any signs of haemorrhage e.g. from umbilicus? Is there scalp swelling suggestive of subaponeurotic haemorrhage?	Obtain access e.g. IV cannula, Umbilical venous catheter (UVC), Intraosseous needle Control visible bleeding Blood samples for first line investigations including blood gas, blood sugar, full blood count, urea and electrolytes and blood culture Consider a fluid bolus 10-20 mL kg^{-1} of 0.9% sodium chloride Consider ordering blood products Give antibiotics Reassess
D	Disability (conscious level)	Assess level of consciousness – Alert – Responsive to stimuli – Unresponsive to all stimuli Check blood glucose Examine pupil size Feel anterior fontanelle and feel the scalp – is there massive swelling crossing the suture lines suggestive of subaponeurotic bleeding? Assess tone, posture and movements	Give 2.5 mL kg^{-1} 10% dextrose IV if indicated Reconsider ABC in infant in light of conscious level Reassess
E	Exposure	Measure the core temperature Undress infant completely and examine front and back and top to bottom Look for evidence blood loss, skin lesions or wounds	Consider warming or cooling Aim for normothermia unless therapeutic hypothermia is indicated Reassess
F	Family	Check the parents understanding and review family history, particularly of feeding, positioning prior to collapse, congenital heart disease, metabolic disorders or consanguinity	Explain honestly about what you have found and your treatment plans are

When should resuscitation be stopped?

An ILCOR systematic review considered the evidence around prolonged resuscitation of newborn infants. Although the available evidence is of very low certainty, they were able to make the following comments and give a weak recommendation.

> "Failure to achieve return of spontaneous circulation in newborn infants despite 10 to 20 min of intensive resuscitation is associated with a high risk of mortality and a high risk of moderate-to-severe neurodevelopmental impairment among survivors.
>
> However, there is no evidence that any specific duration of resuscitation consistently predicts mortality or moderate-to-severe neurodevelopmental impairment. If, despite provision of all the recommended steps of resuscitation and excluding reversible causes, a newborn infant requires on-going cardiopulmonary resuscitation (CPR) after birth, we suggest discussion of discontinuing resuscitative efforts with the clinical team and family. A reasonable time frame to consider this change in goals of care is around 20 min after birth."

The difficulty of this decision-making emphasises the need for senior help to be sought as soon as possible.

Considerations post resuscitation

Infants who are successfully resuscitated will need admission to a neonatal intensive care unit. Transfer to an appropriate centre may be required, for example for therapeutic hypothermia, ongoing intensive care or specialist input e.g. cardiology, surgical or metabolic treatment.

Communication with parents

SUPC is particularly shocking for parents as by definition it follows a period of perceived normality. Parents often feel guilty for not recognising their baby's deterioration sooner or may feel responsible for the collapse, especially if the baby was breastfeeding or having skin to skin contact. A team member should be allocated support and communicate with parents during their baby's resuscitation and inform them clearly of the outcome and ongoing plans. Communication must be factual, clear and honest and avoid speculation.

The remainder of this chapter will briefly outline management of specific causes of SUPC. In all causes, the initial approach will be as outlined above following the sequential ABCDEF approach.

Hypoglycaemia

Hypoglycaemia is common in the term newborn infant. A widely accepted, although commonly debated, definition of hypoglycaemia is a blood glucose level < 2.6 mmol L^{-1}.

Wherever possible, blood glucose should be measured using a specific blood glucose analyser or blood gas machine.

However, bedside stick reagent tests are often used on the postnatal wards. These tend to over read and a low result must always be followed by confirmatory test.

There is evidence of a significant risk of morbidity, including long term neurodevelopmental problems associated with sustained hypoglycaemia in ill or symptomatic babies.

There are well recognised risk factors for developing neonatal hypoglycaemia which include:

- intrauterine growth restriction / small for gestational age
- prematurity
- maternal diabetes (gestational or pre-existing)
- maternal medication including Beta-blockers, oral hypoglycaemic agents
- sepsis
- perinatal asphyxia / HIE
- polycythaemia
- hypothermia.

In addition, hypoglycaemia can be the result of various endocrine, genetic and metabolic conditions.

Many cases of hypoglycaemia can be anticipated and monitoring of pre-feed glucose levels with careful enteral feeding regimens can prevent significant hypoglycaemia. Breast feeding should be encouraged wherever possible.

Infants with hypoglycaemia may be asymptomatic or may exhibit irregular respiration, apnoea, hypotonia, poor suck, irritability, jitteriness, lethargy or seizures. A blood sugar level must form part of the immediate assessment of any unwell baby.

Treatment of hypoglycaemia

- Initially a bolus of 2.5 mL kg^{-1} of 10% dextrose should be given intravenously followed by a continuous dextrose infusion.
- If hypoglycaemia persists then increasing concentrations of IV Dextrose must be given (12.5% dextrose can be given safely peripherally, for higher concentrations central access must be obtained).
- In refractive hypoglycaemia or where there is difficulty obtaining IV or IO access, treatment with glucagon (SC, IV or IM) can be given followed by a glucose infusion. Infants of diabetic mothers may require high doses of glucagon.

- Oral glucose gels have been used in babies where IV access is difficult.
- Always consider an underlying cause for the hypoglycaemia.

There is a national framework for practice for management of hypoglycaemia in the full term infant published by NHS Improvement and BAPM in 2017.

The blue or grey baby

It is not uncommon in the postnatal period for staff to express concern that a baby appears blue or grey. Cyanosis becomes visible when there is an excess of deoxygenated haemoglobin in the blood. The degree of cyanosis and blue discolouration of the skin will depend on the baby's oxygen saturation and haemoglobin concentration. Cyanosis is more visible in the polycythaemic infant compared with an anaemic infant. A grey discolouration of the skin is a worrying sign and may represent cyanosis or shock (Table 12.4). If there is any doubt, pre and post-ductal oxygen saturations should be measured.

Cyanosis may be central or peripheral. Peripheral cyanosis is present in the extremities and may be a result of normal postnatal adaptation or a physiological response to cold. It can also result from vasoconstriction (e.g. in sepsis).

Increasing or spreading peripheral cyanosis should alert you to an underlying pathology. Central cyanosis is manifested by blue/grey discolouration of the centrally perfused areas such as the mucous membranes inside the mouth.

Cyanosis and hypoxia are the result of inadequate functioning of either the heart or the lungs. There may be a primary heart or lung problem or cyanosis could be secondary to other problems e.g. sepsis.

Table 12.4 Potential causes of cyanosis/pallor

Respiratory	Respiratory distress syndrome, pneumonia, meconium aspiration syndrome, persistent pulmonary hypertension of the newborn (PPHN), pneumothorax, congenital abnormalities (e.g. congenital diaphragmatic hernia or cystic adenomatoid malformation of the lung).
Cardiac	Congenital cyanotic heart disease (e.g. transposition of the great arteries, total anomalous pulmonary venous drainage, tricuspid atresia, tetralogy of Fallot, truncus arteriosus, critical pulmonary stenosis). Critical obstruction to the systemic circulation will cause pallor/greyness (e.g. aortic stenosis, hypoplastic left heart).
CNS disease	Intra/periventricular haemorrhage, meningitis, seizures causing hypoventilation.
Other	Polycythaemia, sepsis, shock, methaemoglobinaemia.

Treatment of cyanosis/pallor

Follow the ARNI approach; particular attention must be paid to identifying potentially life-threatening or worrying features. Things to consider in your assessment are:

A B Airway and breathing

- Respiratory distress makes a respiratory aetiology more likely.
- Check for pneumothorax and if present clinically consider the need for cold light examination, needle aspiration or chest drain insertion.
- Order a chest X-ray early.
- If PPHN is suspected (e.g. with a history of meconium aspiration) manage as discussed in Chapter 8 including considering inhaled Nitric Oxide if available.

C Circulation

- Is there a murmur? Are the pulses normal?
- Cyanosis associated with a murmur or abnormal pulses make a cardiac lesion more likely.
- If pulses are diminished consider critically obstructed systemic circulation (coarctation of the aorta, aortic stenosis, hypoplastic left heart) or severe sepsis.
- Measure pre and post-ductal saturations and perform a blood gas.
- Consider if a formal cardiac assessment is needed including echocardiogram; discuss with cardiology team.
- Consider starting prostaglandin (see Chapter 8).

There should be a low threshold for starting prostaglandin in an unwell infant. Consider starting prostaglandin if:

- there is a murmur and cyanosis
- if the infant has reduced pulses
- the patient is critically unwell.

D Disability

- Are there signs of neurological compromise?
- What is the blood sugar?
- Is the baby having seizures?

A blue or grey baby is likely to have a very significant underlying pathology and will need rapid assessment and management as described above to treat potentially life-threatening problems and will need ongoing definitive care.

Sepsis

Newborn infants are vulnerable to infection. The risk of a significant bacterial infection is at its highest in the newborn period than at any other time in life. Sepsis must always be considered in an infant with an unexpected collapse. Most postnatal collapse from sepsis is the result of early onset sepsis as discussed in Chapter 10.

Prompt administration of appropriate antibiotics improves survival. Infants with significant sepsis may need repeated fluid boluses.

Any infant who collapses on the postnatal ward should be presumed to be suffering from sepsis and receive broad spectrum antibiotics intravenously pending ongoing definitive diagnosis and care.

Seizures

Seizures are not uncommon in the newborn period (Chapter 11). They are rarely idiopathic and are often a manifestation of serious underlying abnormalities (Table 12.5).

Table 12.5 Common causes of neonatal seizures

Neurological
Hypoxic ischaemic encephalopathy, intracranial haemorrhage (subarachnoid, subdural, intraventricular, periventricular), cerebral infarction, congenital cerebral malformations, central nervous system trauma.
Metabolic abnormalities
Hypoglycaemia, hypocalcaemia, hypomagnesaemia, hypo/hypernatraemia, pyridoxine deficiency.
Infection
Meningitis, sepsis, encephalitis, congenital infection.
Neonatal drug withdrawal
Polycythaemia
Inborn errors of metabolism

It can be difficult to discriminate between jitteriness, benign myoclonic jerks and seizures.

In the jittery infant, eye movements will be normal and the limbs will stop moving if held gently. Isolated jerks of a non-repetitive nature occurring mainly during sleep are likely to be benign.

Neonatal seizures may be subtle and include:
- deviation of the eyes
- repetitive blinking
- lip smacking
- apnoeas
- cycling of the limbs
- generalised tonic / clonic movements.

Investigation and treatment of seizures is covered in Chapter 11.

12: Summary learning

SUPC is a serious potentially life-threatening problem. Rapid early assessment using the ARNI algorithm must be aimed at treating potentially life-threatening problems and trying to improve the clinical situation sufficiently to enable enough time to make a diagnosis and plan definitive care.

My key take-home messages from this chapter are:

Further reading

Becher JC, Bhushan S, Lyon A. Unexpected collapse in apparently healthy newborns – a prospective national study of a missing cohort of neonatal deaths and near death events. Arch Dis Child Fetal Neonatal Ed 2012; 97: F30-34.

Guidelines for the investigation of newborn infants who suffer a sudden and unexpected postnatal collapse in the first week of life. Recommendations from a professional group on sudden unexpected postnatal collapse. British Association of Perinatal Medicine. March 2011.

Identification and Management of Neonatal Hypoglycaemia in the Full Term Infant (2017). A BAPM Framework for Practice. https://www.bapm.org/resources/40-identification-and-management-of-neonatal-hypoglycaemia-in-the-full-term-infant-2017

Penny, DJ, Shekerdemian LS. Management of the neonate with symptomatic congenital heart disease. Arch Dis Child Fetal Neonatal Ed 2001; 84: F141-F145.

Weber MA, Ashworth MT, Risdon RA, Brooke I, Malone M, Sebire NJ. Sudden unexpected neonatal death in the first week of life: autopsy findings from a specialist centre. J Matern Fetal Neonatal Med. 2009 May; 22:3 98-404.

Vergnano S, Menson E, Kennea N et al. Source Neonatal infections in England: the NeonIN surveillance network. Arch Dis Child Fetal Neonatal Ed. 2011; 96(1): F9-F14. Epub 2010 Sep 27.

Practical procedures

13

In this chapter

Neonatal percutaneous central line insertion (long line)

Peripheral arterial line insertion

Umbilical arterial and venous access

Neonatal lumbar puncture

Intraosseous line insertion

Chest drain insertion

The learning outcomes will enable you to:

Be familiar with common neonatal practical procedures

Introduction

Neonatal practical procedures are technically challenging and cannot be learnt from a manual.

This chapter aims to summarise the indications, practical techniques and common complications of some of the more commonly performed practical procedures in neonatal intensive care. Neonatal practical procedures should be learnt at the cot side with direct supervision or practiced in a simulated environment until competence is achieved.

Tracheal intubation and airway adjuncts are discussed in Chapter 7.

Always consider analgesia prior to any practical procedure and remember to document any procedures performed in the medical notes.

Infection prevention

Infection is a serious problem in neonatal intensive care. Catheter-associated blood stream infection is a cause of significant morbidity.

The practical procedures listed in this chapter should be performed using an aseptic non-touch techniques unless the procedure is being performed as a life saving emergency. The operator should wear appropriate personal protective equipment after thoroughly washing their hands.

Skin should be prepared in line with national guidelines using chlorhexidine and alcohol skin disinfectant. Care should be taken to avoid skin burns from residual alcohol especially on delicate preterm skin. Surgical drapes should be used, and care should be taken not to contaminate the sterile field.

For each practical procedure the following are discussed:
- indications for the procedure
- practical tips and advice
- common complications and how to avoid them.

For every practical procedure all the equipment should be prepared and set out in advance. Remember that help may be required and many procedures require two people. All procedures should be appropriately documented in line with national safety standards.

Neonatal percutaneous central line insertion (long line)

Indication

Intravenous access for:
- Total Parenteral Nutrition (TPN)
- Medications (e.g. inotropes)
- Solutions with high concentrations of glucose or electrolytes.

Technique

1. Identify a large vein for the site of insertion (e.g. long saphenous vein, medial antebrachial vein, cubital vein, accessory cephalic vein, superficial temporal vein).
2. Determine the length of the catheter to be inserted by measuring from the site of insertion to the xiphoid for the leg and sternal angle for the arm.
3. Prime the catheter lumen with 0.9% sodium chloride.
4. Clean the identified leg or arm with the skin preparation and let it dry for 30 s – 1 min. The whole limb should be cleaned, from groin to toes, or armpit to finger tips around the whole circumference.
5. To prevent chemical burns, clean away the antiseptic solution with 0.9% sodium chloride and let the limb dry fully.
6. Place the sterile towels around the site of insertion and leave the leg or arm accessible for the procedure by placing it through a hole in a sterile towel.
7. Identify the vein and insert the needle or introducer into the vein until there is a good flash back of blood.
8. Using non-toothed forceps, thread the catheter slowly 1–2 mm at a time, until the desired length is inserted. Sometimes the threading of the catheter into the vein can be difficult. Be patient and keep advancing the catheter slowly until the 5 cm mark is achieved. Once the 5 cm mark is reached, the catheter is making its way into the vein. Continue to insert it until the desired length is achieved.
9. Flush the catheter slowly with 0.9% sodium chloride to ensure patency and then connect to an infusion running slowly (1 mL h) pending confirmation of position.
10. Some catheters have a guide wire which should be removed.
11. Use the gauze swab to press the catheter at the site of entry and remove the introducer.
12. Press until bleeding stops. This may take up to 10–15 min.
13. Secure the catheter. The insertion site should remain clearly visible.
14. Apply an occlusive dressing to cover the site. Ensure the catheter and the catheter hub are completely covered.
15. Perform an X-ray to determine the position of the catheter tip. Contrast is not usually required.

Neonatal Seldinger central venous lines are now available.

Complications	
Catheter infection	Use strict aseptic non-touch technique.
Misplaced catheter	Ensure that the catheter tip position is confirmed radiologically. Rarely, long line tips in the right atrium can cause cardiac tamponade, these lines should be pulled back to avoid this serious complication. Rare cases of percutaneous catheters inserted via the lower limbs inadvertently entering the lumbar vein.
Bleeding	Apply firm pressure to the site prior to dressing.

Insertion of an intraosseous line

Indication

- Intraosseous lines have been used as emergency access in the event of failed venous/umbilical access. They are not commonly used in neonatal intensive care but are a backup option for emergency vascular access in resuscitation.
- All neonatal resuscitation drugs and emergency fluids can be administered down an intraosseous line.

Technique

1. There are different types of intraosseous line – newer types are inserted using an automatic 'drill.'
2. Identify the insertion point on the anteromedial surface of the tibia, just below the tibial tuberosity.
3. Insert the needle applying downwards pressure until a 'give' is felt and the needle enters the bone marrow cavity.
4. Take any samples needed (notify the lab that they are bone marrow samples). Prioritise important samples such as glucose and cultures.

Complications
Intraosseous lines should not be used if the bone is abnormal, e.g. osteogenesis imperfecta.
There is risk of fracture to the bone particularly in small babies.
Bone marrow embolism has been described.

Umbilical line insertion

Indication

Venous line
- Emergency access for resuscitation drugs.
- Administration of medications, e.g. inotropes and TPN.
- Monitoring of central venous pressure.
- Performing an exchange transfusion.

Arterial line
- Monitoring of arterial blood pressure.
- Arterial blood gas sampling.
- For performing an exchange transfusion.

Technique

1. For a non-emergency line, full aseptic non-touch technique should be used.
2. Prime the umbilical line with 0.9% sodium chloride and measure how far you wish to insert it. One method of estimating the length of insertion is:
   Venous line – distance from the umbilicus to the xiphisternum + the length of remaining cord
   Arterial line – distance from umbilicus to left shoulder + the length of the cord
3. Identify the umbilical vessels – there is one vein, and usually 2 arteries and check for cord abnormalities. The vein is thin walled and often bleeds when the cord is cut. The arteries are smaller and have thicker walls.
4. Tie a ligature around the base of the cord to control bleeding.
5. Grasp the cord with artery forceps to secure it.
6. Dilate the vessel with a pair of fine forceps or an umbilical dilator. The artery will usually need more dilatation than the vein.
7. Pass the catheter into the umbilical vessel – resistance is often felt at the umbilical ring.
8. Advance to the appropriate length – blood should be easy to aspirate.
9. Secure the catheter according to local policy.
10. X-ray to assess umbilical catheter position.
    Suitable venous position: in the ductus venous or inferior vena cava but outside the heart
    Suitable arterial position: high position thoracic vertebra 6 (T6 –T8) low position below second lumbar vertebra (L2).

Complications	
Catheter associated infection	Use strict aseptic non-touch technique.
Compromised perfusion	Always check the perfusion of the legs and buttocks after arterial line insertion.
Haemorrhage	Especially if a line is accidentally displaced. Always use a transducer as this may alert you to accidental disconnection.
Air embolus	Use appropriate catheter bungs and do not leave a venous open to the air.

Peripheral arterial line insertion

Indication

- Continuous monitoring of invasive blood pressure
- Accurate measurement of blood gases
- To perform an exchange transfusion

Technique

1. Identify the artery – suitable sites include radial and posterior tibial arteries. Ulnar, brachial and femoral arteries can be used but are higher risk because they have no back up blood supply if that artery is occluded or damaged. A fibreoptic cold light can make identification easier.
2. Prior to insertion, check perfusion of the limb using Allen's test which is where both the radial and ulnar arteries are occluded with fingertip pressure then the ulnar is released. A normal result is when the pallor of the hand resolves through perfusion from the ulnar artery. A negative test suggests poor perfusion from the ulnar artery meaning radial arterial line insertion is more likely to cause hand ischaemia. Do not use a limb where there has been a recent arterial line.
3. Palpate the point of maximal pulsation of the artery.
4. Insert the cannula into the artery aiming towards the point of maximal pulsation. Attempt to puncture the centre of the artery through the anterior wall at an angle of 30 degrees.
5. Once a flashback of blood is seen, advance the needle slightly, and then holding the needle still, advance the catheter. Remove the needle. There should be pulsatile blood flow.
6. It may be helpful to flush with 0.9% sodium chloride to distend the artery while advancing the cannula.
7. Attach the cannula to the arterial connector and 3 way Luer lock tap and slowly flush with 0.9% sodium chloride. An arterial line should always be attached to a pressure transducer.
8. Apply an occlusive dressing and tape the catheter and extension line in place. Confirm perfusion of the distal limb.

Complications	
Compromised perfusion	Always examine the fingers/toes, checking for colour and perfusion. This should be assessed regularly whilst the arterial line is in place.
Bleeding	A disconnected line can result in significant haemorrhage. Always use an arterial transducer as the loss of trace will alert you to possible problems.

Seldinger chest drain insertion

Technique

1. Prepare the chest using standard aseptic non-touch technique. Ideally, infiltrate the insertion area with local anaesthetic (1 mL 1% lidocaine); this will take a few minutes to work.
2. Identify the insertion point. (above 5th rib, in 4th–5th intercostal space, mid to anterior axillary line.
   Safety point: double check side that the chest drain needs to be inserted.
3. Attach a 5 mL or 10 mL syringe to the needle and gently advance the needle through the chest wall, aspirating the syringe as the needle is advanced. Air will be aspirated as the needle is advanced into the pleural space.
4. Remove the syringe and attach the wire introducer and guide wire to the needle. (The guide wire lies within a sterility sleeve).
5. Holding the needle in place, gently advance the guide wire into the chest cavity; there should be little resistance. Hold the guide wire in place and remove the needle and sterility sleeve, leaving the guide wire in place.
6. Feed the dilator over the guide wire and gently advance through the chest wall, making a dilated track, then remove the dilator. The operator should be in control of the guidewire at all times.
7. Slide the chest drain over the guide wire and advance through the dilated track into the chest cavity. All the holes at the tip of the drain should be inside the chest cavity.
8. Hold the drain in place and remove the guide wire. Attach the adaptor to the drain. The end of the collection tubing may require cutting to fit the adaptor.
9. Many drains are pig-tailed and do not routinely require stitching in place; it can be held in place with a clear adhesive dressing against the chest wall. Straight chest drains are also available and may require more careful securing.

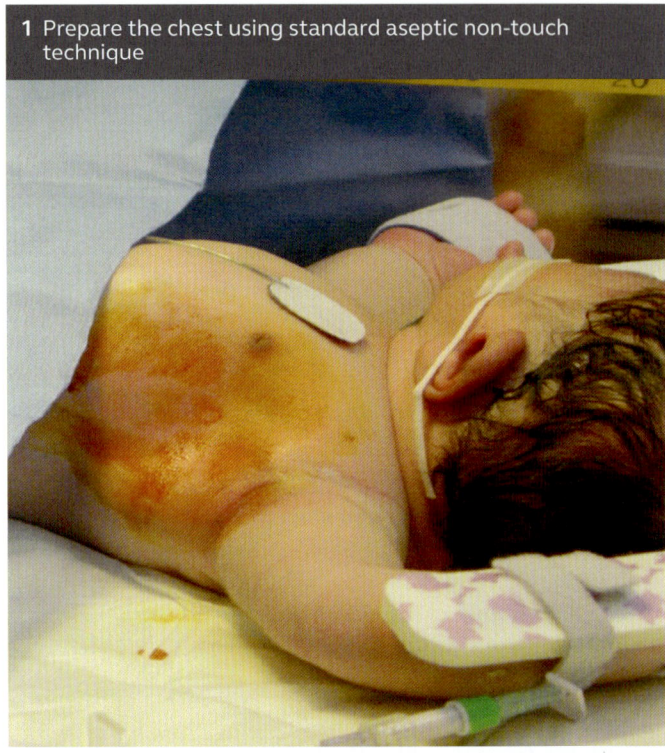

1 Prepare the chest using standard aseptic non-touch technique

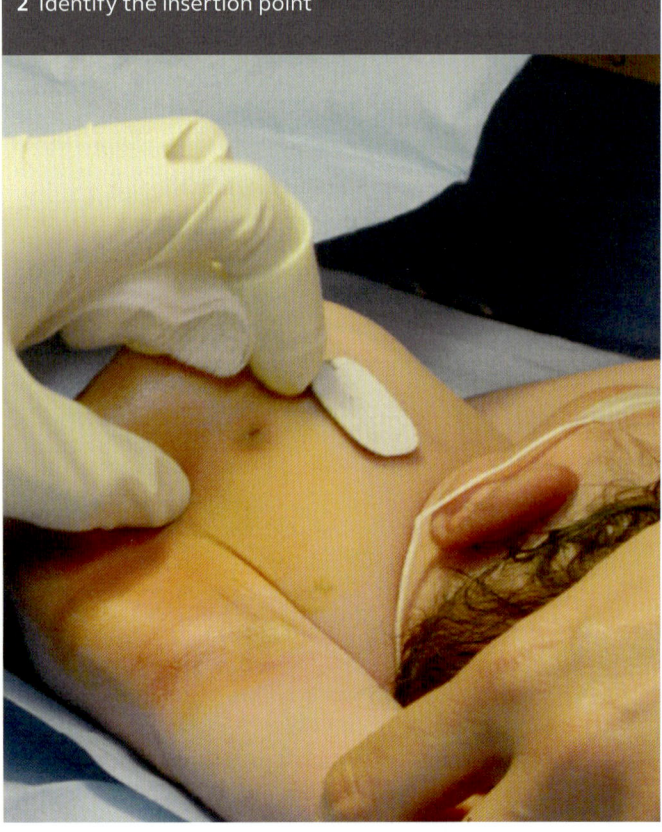

2 Identify the insertion point

3 Attach a 5 mL or 10 mL syringe to the needle and gently advance the needle through the chest wall

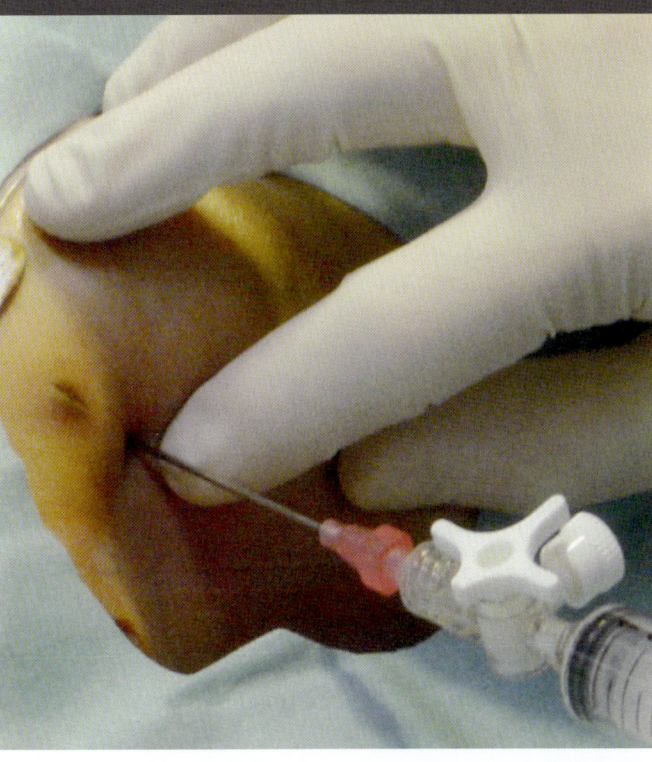

4 Remove the syringe and attach the wire introducer and guide wire to the needle

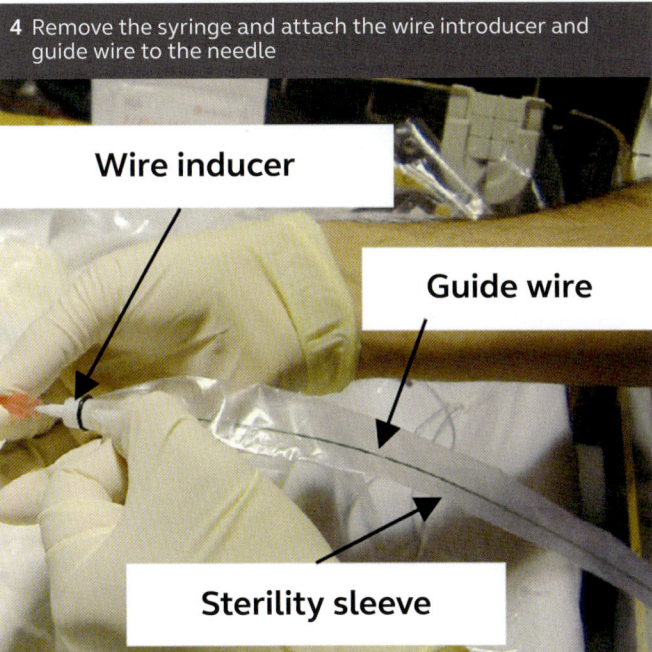

Wire inducer
Guide wire
Sterility sleeve

7 Slide the chest drain over the guide wire and advance through the dilated track into the chest cavity

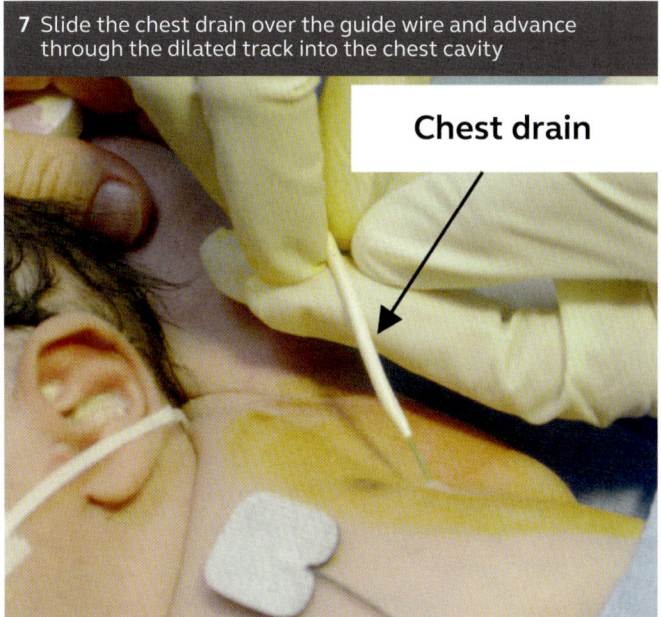

Chest drain

9 Many drains are pig-tailed and do not routinely require stitching in place

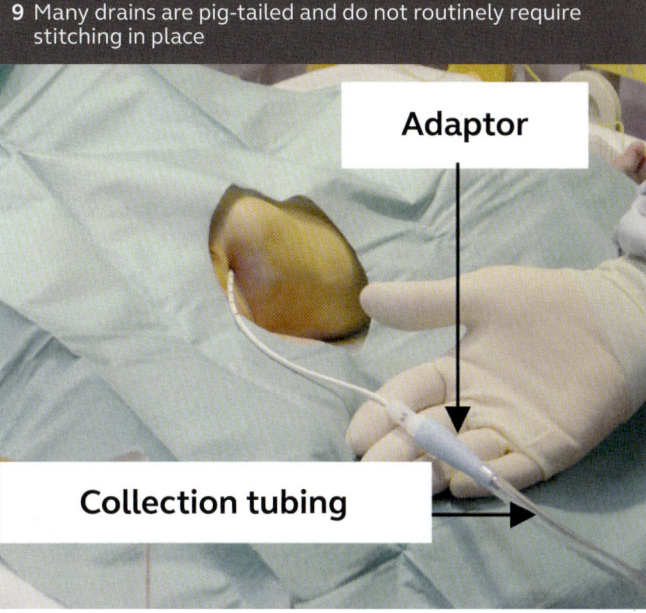

Adaptor
Collection tubing

ARNI   Resuscitation Council UK   Practical procedures   113

13 Surgical chest drain insertion

Technique

1. Use a sterile non-touch technique.
2. Clean the skin over the area in which drain is to be inserted.
3. The landmarks for insertion are either laterally; the 5th or 6th intercostal space in the anterior axillary line, or rarely anteriorly; the 2nd intercostal space in the mid-clavicular line.
4. Take care to avoid the nipple and breast bud area.
5. Infiltrate the skin with local anaesthetic (1 mL 1% lidocaine) or give a small dose of analgesia; wait for it to take effect.
6. Make a small incision in the skin and intercostal muscles above the rib at the selected site. Separate the muscle fibres using fine blunt forceps until you see the pleura (a shiny grey membrane).
7. Pierce the pleura and enter the pleural space using the fine blunt artery forceps.
8. Remove the trocar from the chest drain and insert the flexible chest drain along the line of the tract (you may need to grasp the end using the artery forceps).
9. Insert the drain 3–5 cm, aiming anteriorly and superiorly to drain air, or posteriorly to drain fluid.
10. Connect the drain to the underwater seal. The drain should bubble and the fluid level will move with respiration.
11. Secure the chest drain by stitching into place with a suture. Tie the suture around the chest tube tightly. Do not put a 'purse string' suture around the entry site as this can cause scarring.
12. Secure to the chest-wall using steristrips and a clear adhesive dressing.
13. Order an urgent chest X-ray to check position of drain and ensure adequate evacuation of air.
14. After inserting the drain ensure that the tubing is secured to a fixed site (e.g. baby's mattress) to prevent accidental dislodgement.
15. Document the procedure fully in the patient's notes.

Removal of a chest drain

1. Confirm that the reason for the chest drain insertion has resolved.
2. Remember that a recurrence of pneumothorax is more likely if the baby is receiving positive pressure support.
3. Remove drain and rapidly close the incision with steristrips. If the wound is gaping and cannot be closed with wound closure strips use one or two interrupted stitches.
4. Observe carefully for 24 h. If symptoms recur, recheck ABC and repeat CXR.

Complications
Complications of chest drain insertion include damage to intra thoracic structures from guidewires or drains, haemorrhage and infection.
Some neonatologists prefer to insert a chest drain immediately, rather than performing a needle thoracocentesis.
Take care to avoid the breast bud area as a scar in this area can lead to later disfigurement.

Emergency needle thoracocentesis

Indication

Drainage of pneumothorax or fluid in the chest cavity.

Pneumothorax can be confirmed by transillumination (cold light examination) (Figure 13.1) or chest X-ray (Figure 13.2).

Technique for needle thoracocentesis

1. Insert a butterfly needle or cannula in the second intercostal space, in the midclavicular line perpendicular to the chest.
2. Insert the needle just above the rib and aspirate with a syringe until you get air.
3. Hold the end of the butterfly needle under water or attach a 3-way tap to aspirate the air.
4. Once stabilised, consider insertion of a formal chest drain.
5. Leaving the needle in the thorax once the lung has reinflated can lead to serious damage to the lung tissue.

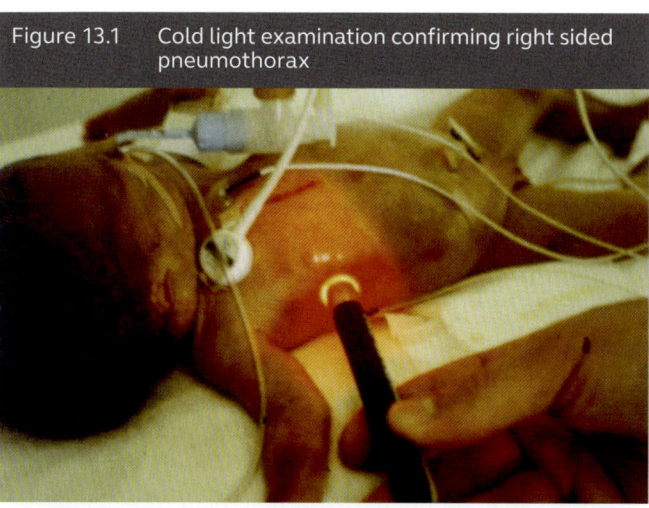

Figure 13.1 Cold light examination confirming right sided pneumothorax

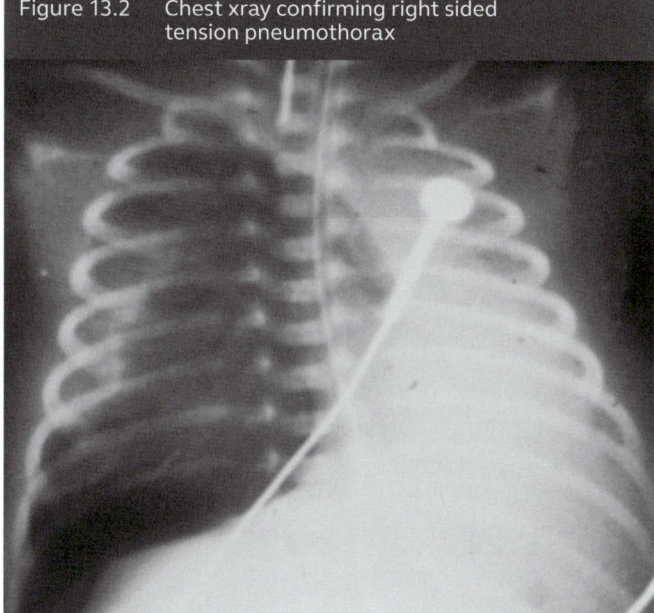

Figure 13.2 Chest xray confirming right sided tension pneumothorax

Lumbar puncture (LP)

Indication

- Diagnosis of meningitis
- Treatment of post haemorrhagic hydrocephalus
- To measure CSF pressure

Technique

1. Position the baby in a lateral position, held with the hips and neck flexed to open up the spaces between the vertebrae. A sitting position is also possible.
2. Full aseptic non-touch technique should be used.
3. Identify your landmarks – a vertical line joining the posterior superior iliac spines will pass through the L 3/4 disc space.
4. Insert an appropriate size lumbar puncture needle (usually 20 G or 22 G) in the midline.
5. The needle will pass through the spinous ligament and you will feel a 'give' as it enters the subarachnoid space to obtain CSF for neurometabolic investigations.
6. Remove the stylet and collect the CSF as it drips out.
7. If there is no CSF, advance the needle slightly forward until flow is seen.
8. Samples should be sent for microbiology and biochemical evaluation and if necessary virology or other investigations as indicated.
9. Remove the needle and apply a sterile dressing.

Complications
LP should not be performed if there are signs of raised intracranial pressure as there is a risk of coning. This is a low risk in infants as the fontanelle is open.
Low platelets and severe coagulopathy are contraindications to LP.
Babies with haemodynamic instability may not tolerate the procedure.

Further reading

Cable DG, Mullany CJ, Schaff HV. The Allen test. Ann of Thorac Surg. 1999: 67: 876-877.

Massaro AN, Rais-Bahrami K. Peripheral artery cannulation. Ch3. in: MacDonald MG, Ramasethu J. Atlas of Procedures in Neonatology. 5th Ed. Lippincott, Williams & Wilkins. Philadelphia. 2012. pp. 182-193.

Pearse RG. Percutaneous catheterisation of the radial artery in newborn babies using transillumination. Arch Dis Childhood. 1978; 53: 549-554.

Rais-Bahrami K, MacDonald MG. Thoracostomy. Ch38. in: MacDonald MG, Ramasethu J. Atlas of Procedures in Neonatology. 5th Ed. Lippincott, Williams & Wilkins. Philadelphia. 2012. pp. 255-272.

Said MM, Rais-Bahrami K. Endotracheal intubation. Ch36. in: MacDonald MG, Ramasethu J. Atlas of Procedures in Neonatology. 5th Ed. Lippincott, Williams & Wilkins. Philadelphia. 2012. pp. 236-249.

Said MM, Rais-Bahrami K. Umbilical artery cannulation. Ch29. in: MacDonald MG, Ramasethu J. Atlas of Procedures in Neonatology. 5th Ed. Lippincott, Williams & Wilkins. Philadelphia. 2012. pp. 156-172.

Said MM, Rais-Bahrami K. Umbilical venous cannulation. Ch30. in: MacDonald MG, Ramasethu J. Atlas of Procedures in Neonatology. 5th Ed. Lippincott, Williams & Wilkins. Philadelphia. 2012. pp. 173-181.

Woods SL. Lumbar puncture. Ch17. in: MacDonald MG, Ramasethu J. Atlas of Procedures in Neonatology. 5th Ed. Lippincott, Williams & Wilkins. Philadelphia. 2012. pp. 104-108.

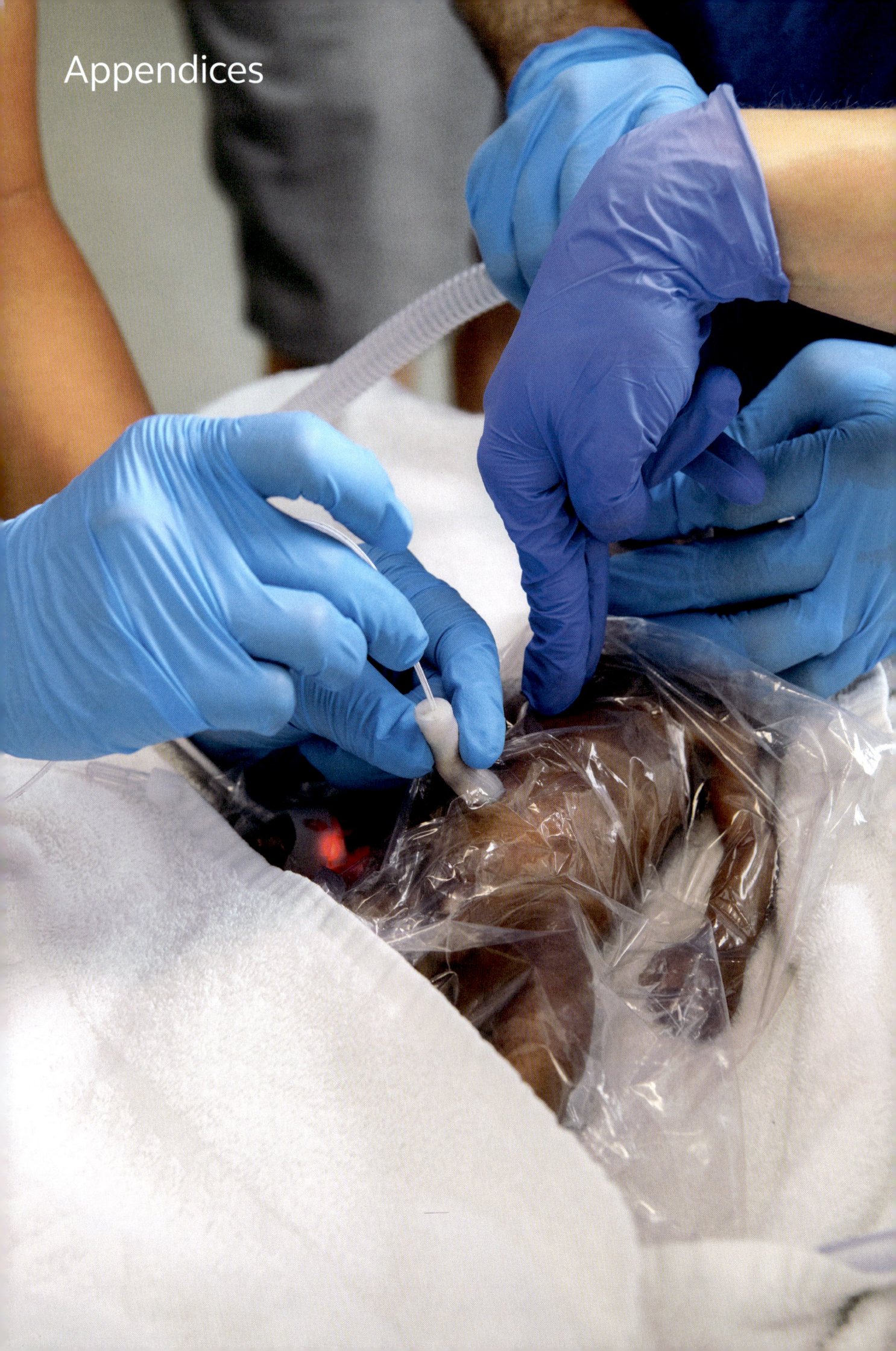

Appendices

Appendix A
Interpreting blood gases

Introduction

Correct interpretation of capillary and arterial blood gas measurements is a key component in the early care and stabilisation of a baby on the neonatal unit. It is important to be able to identify respiratory and metabolic problems so that appropriate actions can be taken.

In babies, blood gases can be measured in a number of ways:

Arterial
This is the gold standard. Sick babies on a neonatal unit often have an indwelling arterial line to allow for regular accurate assessment of blood gases. However, arterial lines can lead to complications, particularly in the smallest babies.

Capillary
In babies, capillary blood gas measurement is often used. Capillary gases give a reliable measure of the partial pressure of carbon dioxide, pH, base excess and bicarbonate. The measurement of the partial pressure of oxygen is unreliable.

Capillary gases may not be accurate if there is poor peripheral perfusion or circulatory compromise; an arterial gas is required in this instance.

Venous
Venous blood gas measurement can be used to estimate pH and base excess. They are less useful for measuring and interpreting the partial pressure of oxygen and carbon dioxide.

Central venous gases can be obtained from an indwelling umbilical catheter.

Cord gases
Gases taken from the umbilical artery and vein shortly after birth can be used to measure pH and acid base status. Babies that have suffered from intrapartum hypoxia are often (but not always) acidotic and this information can be used to guide further treatment for instance therapeutic hypothermia (see Chapter 11). The arterial sample reflects the baby's condition and is often the more acidotic than the umbilical venous sample.

Interpretation of neonatal blood gases
There are five pieces of information that are used to interpret a neonatal blood gas. Normal arterial blood gas ranges for a term infant are shown below:

Measurement	Normal range in blood
pH	7.27–7.39
$PaCO_2$ (partial pressure of carbon dioxide kPa)	4.0–5.6
PaO_2 (partial pressure of oxygen kPa)	7.1–12.3
Bicarbonate (mmol/l)	19.2–24.4
Base Excess (mmol/l)	-3 to +3

pH

The acidity or alkalinity of a solution is determined by the concentration of hydrogen ions (H^+). The actual concentration of hydrogen ions in the body is very low, and so the pH scale is often used. The pH scale is a logarithmic scale that expresses hydrogen ion concentration.

A small change in pH represents a much larger change in hydrogen ion concentration.

A low pH indicates acidosis and a high pH indicates alkalosis.

The human body uses a system of 'buffers'. These are chemicals that maintain the pH within normal limits.

Alveolar partial pressure

The partial pressure of a gas is the concentration of that gas in a medium.

At atmospheric pressure, the partial pressure of a gas is the same as the percentage (%) of the gas by volume. Partial pressure is measured in kiloPascals (kPa).

$PaCO_2$

Carbon dioxide is produced as a waste product of respiration. It is transported in the blood, either bound to haemoglobin, proteins or dissolved in the plasma.

When dissolved in water, carbon dioxide reacts to form hydrogen (H^+) and bicarbonate ions (HCO_3^-).

$$CO_2 + H_2O \rightleftharpoons H^+ + HCO_3^-$$

Increasing the amount of CO_2 will drive this reaction to the right and increase the production of hydrogen and bicarbonate ions. The bicarbonate in the body produced by respiration is a relatively small amount.

Decreasing alveolar ventilation will lead to an increase in carbon dioxide, which will dissolve to produce hydrogen ions.

High carbon dioxide levels therefore lead to a respiratory acidosis.

Increasing alveolar ventilation will lead to a decrease in carbon dioxide, which will produce less hydrogen ions.

Low carbon dioxide levels therefore lead to a respiratory alkalosis.

PaO$_2$

The concentration of oxygen in inspired air is 21% representing a partial pressure of 21 kPa.

The partial pressure in the alveolus is less than this as the air is mixed with expired CO$_2$ and water vapour.

High levels of oxygen can be harmful to all babies but particularly to preterm babies. High levels of inspired oxygen produce toxic free radicals and have been associated with the development of retinopathy of prematurity and chronic lung disease.

The optimal PaO$_2$ for preterm babies is unclear and has been the subject of much research.

Bicarbonate

Bicarbonate is an important buffer. Most bicarbonate in the body is generated by the kidneys. Bicarbonate is used to help excrete acids produced by the body.

Bicarbonate binds with hydrogen ions in the serum to neutralise them, producing carbonic acid (H$_2$CO$_3$).

$$H^+ + HCO_3^- \rightleftharpoons H_2CO_3$$

An increased production of hydrogen ions will drive this reaction to the right.

In the kidney, the reaction is driven to the left; hydrogen ions are produced and can be excreted in the urine.

Sometimes, there is an acute rise in acid levels, particularly when there is poor tissue perfusion or hypoxia leading to a rise in lactic acid. Lactate measurement can be helpful in this circumstance.

If the body's buffer systems fail, a metabolic acidosis will develop. In clinical practice, it is important to look for the cause of a metabolic acidosis, rather than immediately treating with bicarbonate. Poor perfusion may be better treated with improved oxygenation, volume expansion or inotropes for example.

Base excess

This is a measure of the amount of excess acid or base in the blood. It is calculated as the amount of acid or base that would need to be added to normalise the pH. A negative base excess is sometimes referred to as a base deficit.

A large negative number implies a **metabolic acidosis**.

A large positive number implies a **metabolic alkalosis**.

Compensation

From the above, we can see that the body has 2 ways of excreting acid, via the lungs and the kidney.

These systems link up and work together:

$$CO_2 + H_2O \rightleftharpoons H_2CO_3 \rightleftharpoons H^+ + HCO_3^-$$

Lungs Kidney

If the CO$_2$ rises, the equation will move to the right, and hydrogen ions will be formed. This will lead to acidosis.

The body will counter this by producing bicarbonate in the kidney, to bind to the hydrogen ions and drive the equation to the left to restore normality. Bicarbonate levels will increase.

This is known as metabolic compensation.

The production of bicarbonate is not instantaneous. A blood gas is described as 'partially compensated' if the pH remains abnormal, and fully compensated if the pH has been fully normalised.

Interpreting a blood gas – simple steps

Interpreting a blood gas can be daunting to start with. It is best to follow these simple steps:

1. Look at the pH	If the pH is low, there is an acidosis.
	If the pH is high there is an alkalosis.
	The next steps aim to identify the primary problem.
2. Look at the carbon dioxide - does this explain the pH?	A high carbon dioxide with a low pH is a respiratory acidosis.
	A low carbon dioxide with a high pH is a respiratory alkalosis.
	If the carbon dioxide is normal, move to step 3.
3. Look at the Base Excess and Bicarbonate - does this explain the pH?	A large negative base excess and low bicarbonate is a metabolic acidosis.
	A large positive base excess and a high bicarbonate is a metabolic alkalosis.
4. Once you have identified the primary problem, check for compensation.	Remember that the body will compensate for a respiratory acidosis by retaining bicarbonate - bicarbonate levels will be high.
	The body will compensate for a respiratory alkalosis by losing bicarbonate; bicarbonate levels will be decreased.
	The body will compensate for a metabolic acidosis by increasing alveolar ventilation - the CO$_2$ will be decreased.
	The body will compensate for a metabolic alkalosis by decreasing alveolar ventilation - the CO$_2$ will be increased.
	Any blood gas interpretation needs to consider all the parameters, not just the pH.

If a blood gas result looks very unusual and not in keeping with the clinical picture, then it should be repeated.

Interpreting blood gases: some practical examples

Blood gas		Interpretation	Clinical example
pH	7.18	Respiratory acidosis	Neonatal respiratory distress syndrome
CO_2	8.9	There is a low pH, high CO_2 and normal BE and bicarbonate	
BE	-2.0		
Bicarbonate	22		
pH	7.48	Respiratory alkalosis	Preterm baby on a ventilator with excessive ventilation
CO_2	2.9	There is a high pH with low CO_2 and normal BE and bicarbonate	
BE	-2.0		
Bicarbonate	22		
pH	7.10	Metabolic acidosis	Preterm baby with hypotension and poor tissue perfusion
CO_2	4.1	There is a low pH with a negative base excess, low bicarbonate and normal CO_2	
BE	-12		
Bicarbonate	17		
pH	7.25	Partially compensated respiratory acidosis	Neonatal chronic lung disease
CO_2	9.8	There is a low pH with high CO_2 respiratory acidosis. The bicarbonate and base excess have risen in an attempt to compensate	
BE	+6.3		
Bicarbonate	29		
pH	7.10	Partially compensated metabolic acidosis	3-hour old infant with hypoxic ischaemic encephalopathy
CO_2	2.9	There is a low pH with low bicarbonate and a negative base excess-metabolic acidosis. The CO_2 is low in an attempt to compensate	
BE	-12		
Bicarbonate	16		
pH	7.12	Mixed respiratory and metabolic acidosis	2-day old infant with Group B Streptococcus pneumonia and poor perfusion
CO_2	8.3	Low pH with high CO_2 and negative base excess indicating a mixed acidosis	
BE	-9		
Bicarbonate	19		

Pulse oximetry

Pulse oximetry is a vital tool for assessing oxygen status. Both low oxygen saturations and excessive oxygen administration can be harmful to babies.

Pulse oximetry is simple to use, relatively cheap and non-invasive. Pulse oximetry is a useful tool in managing term and preterm babies on delivery suite. The pulse oximeter probe contains light emitting diodes (LEDs) and a photoreceptor. Specific neonatal probes exist, and some saturation monitors have software included to minimise movement artefact.

Light produced by the LEDs is transmitted across the baby's limb and some of the light is absorbed. The ratio of transmitted to absorbed light is used to generate the oxygen saturation reading.

The saturation probe needs to be sited on the right hand to produce pre-ductal saturation measurements.

The relationship between oxygen saturation and partial pressure is demonstrated by the oxygen dissociation curve (Figure A1).

The sinusoidal shape of the curve means that an initial drop in arterial oxygen levels is not accompanied by a drop of similar magnitude in oxygen saturations.

There are some limitations to oxygen saturation measurements.

- Poor tissue perfusion often leads to a poor saturation trace and unreliable readings.
- Movement artefact can prevent accurate oxygen saturation readings.
- High ambient light levels can affect oxygen saturation readings.
- Presence of abnormal haemoglobin e.g. methaemoglobin can lead to error in saturation measurements.
- They are less reliable in the presence of profound anaemia.

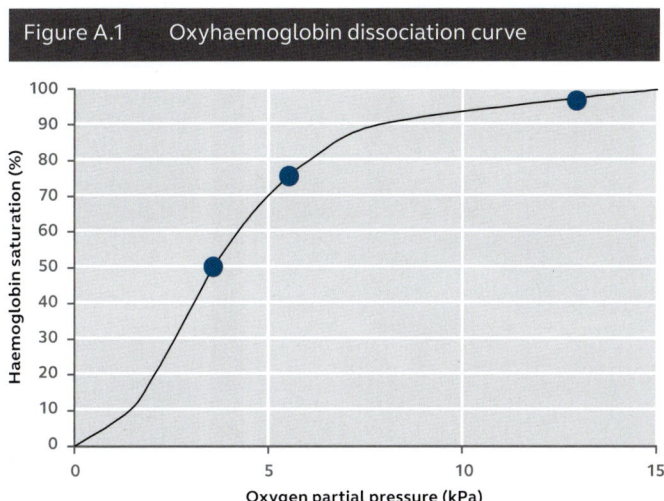

Figure A.1 Oxyhaemoglobin dissociation curve

A: Summary learning

The results of blood gas analysis can be interpreted using a simple stepwise approach.

Look for evidence of compensation.

Treat the baby not the gas: look for the underlying causes of any abnormalities.

Pulse oximetry is a useful tool.

Appendix B
Three key ways to reduce mask leak: 3 P'S

1. Align, roll, check POSITION
Roll the mask onto the face

Align

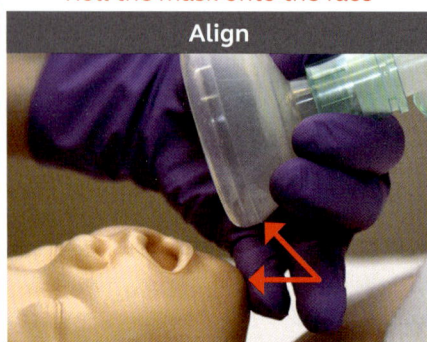

Roll

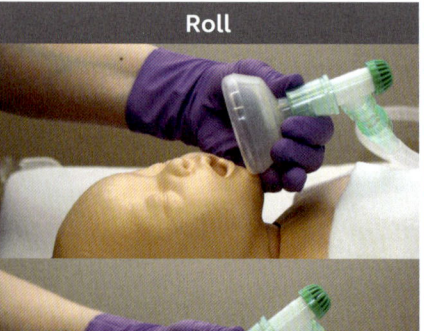

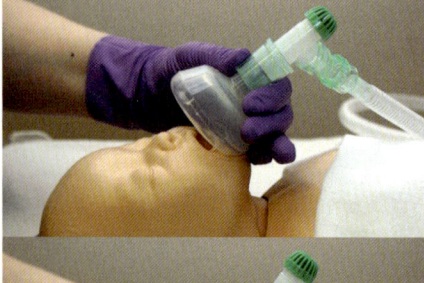

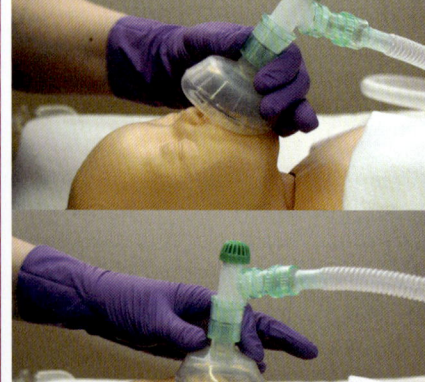

Check POSITION

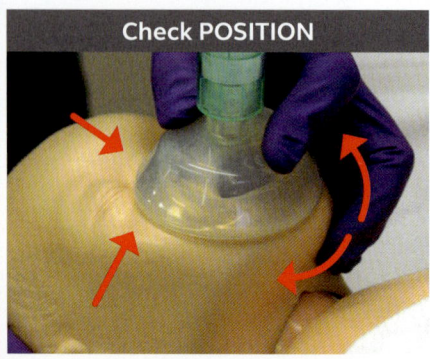

2. Balance the PRESSURE
exerted by the finger and thumb

Two point top hold

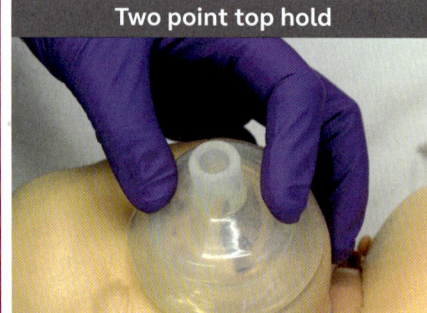

C-grip hold

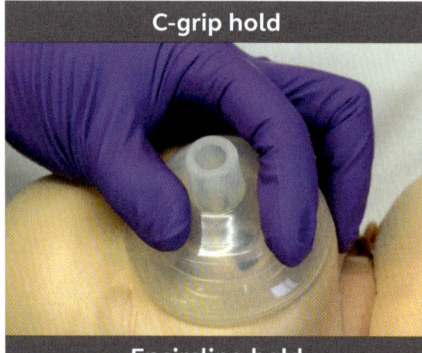

Encircling hold

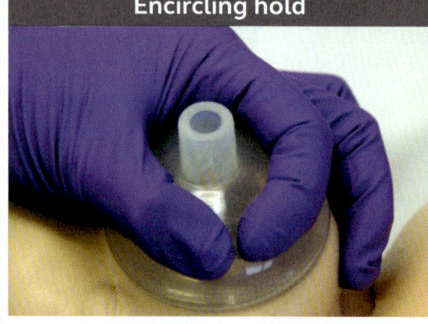

Two handed hold

Two-person hold

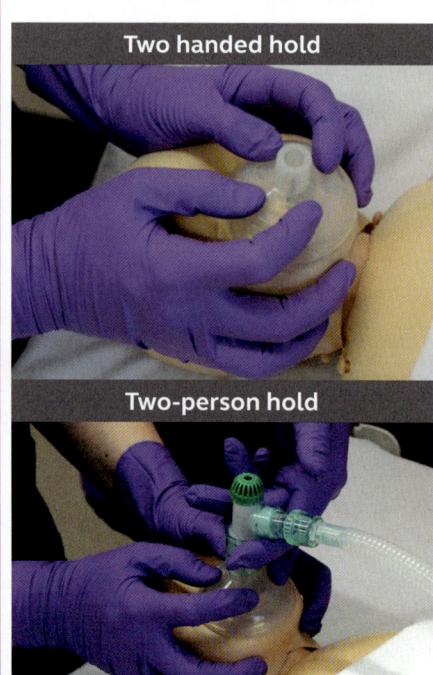

3. PULL the jaw upwards into the mask

Space 3rd to 5th fingers along the mandibular ridge

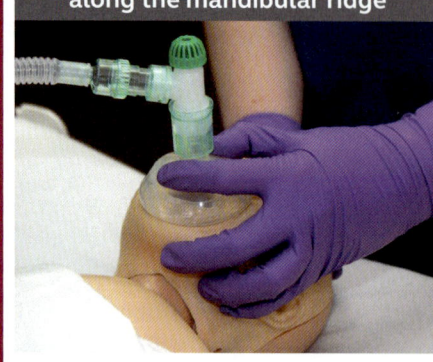

Draw the mandible upwards to provide jaw lift

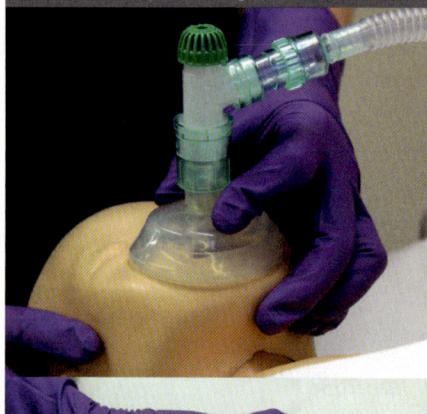

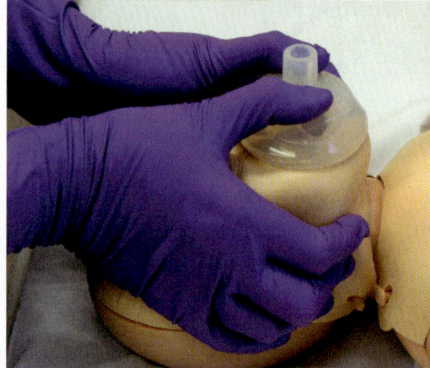

Balance the opposing forces

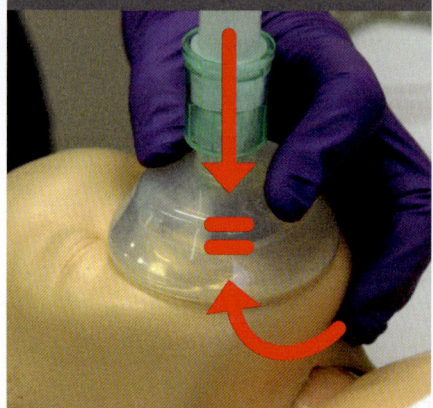

Resuscitation Council UK — ARNI

Appendix C
Personal protective equipment (PPE)

Personal protective equipment

The COVID-19 virus pandemic required careful thought about appropriate levels of PPE needed in resuscitation situations. The need for PPE is not limited to COVID-19 infections as other pathogens can be transmitted in respiratory secretions or blood. The concepts about assessing risk, choosing appropriate PPE and being able to deliver planned resuscitation measures whilst wearing that PPE are generalisable.

Risk assessments

When assessing the risk of transmission of a pathogen to the resuscitation team the following need to be considered:

- Is a specific potentially transmissible pathogen known or suspected in the baby or their mother?
- What is known about the transmissibility of the pathogen?
- Are there concerns about a particular mode of transmission e.g. droplet or aerosol spread from aerosol generating procedures?
- Are there known groups that are more vulnerable to catching or becoming unwell with this pathogen?
- What level of PPE is needed?
- Who is the source of greatest risk, the mother or the baby or both?
- Can exposure be limited by minimising the number in the resuscitation team?
- Where will newborn life support be carried out?
- If post resuscitation care is needed where will this occur, how will the baby be transferred and what isolation or barrier nursing measures are required?

Levels of PPE

Levels of PPE describe increasing amounts of protection and help explain what may be needed in different situations. Exact definitions of levels of PPE may vary but one example is:

Level 1 PPE

- Single pair of gloves
- Disposable plastic apron
- Fluid repellent surgical mask
- Eye protection if you feel there is a risk of patient coughing, or splash or droplet exposure.

Level 2 PPE

- Single pair of gloves
- Long sleeved fluid repellent gown
- FFP3 respirator
- Eye protection (visor which can be disposable or reusable).

FFP3 or equivalent masks do not fit everybody equally well and mask fit testing is advised prior to use in situations with a risk of pathogen transmission. Where required mask fit testing should be done in planned manner in a timely way before being exposed to resuscitation situations with a risk of infection transmission.

Availability of PPE needs to be considered when planning resuscitation services.

Aerosol generating procedures (AGPs)

For pathogens that may be transmitted by aerosolisation and possibly those spread by droplets, AGPs represent a risk of transmission to the resuscitation team. Neonatal AGPs include:

- Mask ventilation
- CPAP
- Intubation
- Ventilation via a tracheal tube or laryngeal mask
- Suctioning of the airway.

Neonatal chest compressions may be an AGP but practically one of the interventions above that are AGPs should always precede the delivery of chest compressions.

Manikin particle dispersal studies show reduced particle dispersal with a high efficiency particulate air (HEPA) filter in place. The filter adds a slight increased resistance to airflow which potentially could increase if the filter is wet for example with longer term use. A filter could be used with either ventilation via a mask or tracheal tube using either a T-piece or bag/valve system. If a filter is used, it is important that it an appropriate size for the baby and does not compromise ventilation. If mask ventilating with a filter in place, care should be taken that the weight of the filter does not affect mask hold and increase mask leak.

Practical use of PPE

The practical difficulties behind the safe donning and doffing of PPE should be considered and standard operating procedures and designated areas can help. The logistics of what PPE a resuscitation team needs and whether a full team needs to be present from the start or whether additional team members join, if needed, should be planned in advance. The additional cognitive load and communication difficulties imposed by wearing higher levels of PPE should not be underestimated. Simulation training can be useful in preparing resuscitation teams for these situations.

Useful links

Resuscitation Council UK Guidelines
Read all of the 2021 guidelines:
resus.org.uk/rcukgl21
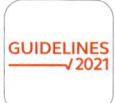

Lifesaver and Lifesaver VR apps
Teach your friends and family lifesaving skills anytime, anywhere:
resus.org.uk/rcuklifesaver
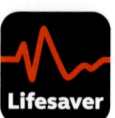

iResus app
Get RCUK guidelines on the go:
resus.org.uk/rcukiresus
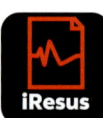

e-Lifesaver
Bring lifesaving training to your non-clinical staff:
resus.org.uk/rcukworkplace
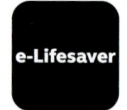

Resuscitation Council UK courses
See all of the courses available:
resus.org.uk/rcukcourses

Follow us on Twitter
@ResusCouncilUK
twitter.com/ResusCouncilUK
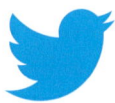

RCUK membership
Get involved and join our community:
resus.org.uk/rcukmembers

Like us on Facebook
facebook.com/ResuscitationCouncilUK
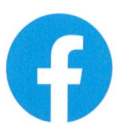

Notes

Notes

Notes

Notes